Care Planning
Pocket Guide

D1363799

Janet Reiss Lederer, RN, MN
Staff Development Instructor
El Camino Hospital Nursing Service
Mountain View, California

Gail L. Marculescu, RN, MSNc
Staff Nurse III—Surgical Unit
El Camino Hospital Nursing Service
Mountain View, California

Judy Gallagher, RN, MS
Head Nurse, Orthopedic Unit
El Camino Hospital Nursing Service
Mountain View, California

Pamela Mills, RN
Staff Nurse, Maternity Unit
El Camino Hospital Nursing Service
Mountain View, California

Care Planning
Pocket Guide

A Nursing Diagnosis Approach

Janet Reiss Lederer, RN, MN

Gail L. Marculescu, RN, MSNc

Judy Gallagher, RN, MS

Pamela Mills, RN

ADDISON-WESLEY PUBLISHING COMPANY
Health Sciences Division, Menlo Park, California
Reading, Massachusetts • Don Mills, Ontario • Wokingham, UK
Amsterdam • Sydney • Singapore • Tokyo • Mexico City
Bogota • Santiago • San Juan

Sponsoring Editor: Katherine Pitcoff
Production Supervisor: Judith Johnstone
Copy Editor: Antonio Padial
Cover Designer: Paul Quin
Cover Illustrator: George Omura
Interior Designer: Paul Quin
Compositor: John Hammett

Addison-Wesley Publishing Company
Health Sciences Division
2725 Sand Hill Road
Menlo Park, California 94025

Library of Congress Cataloging-in-Publication Data
Main Entry under title:
Care planning pocket guide.
      Includes index.
      1. Nursing care plans—Handbooks, manuals, etc.
2. Diagnosis—Handbooks, manuals, etc.   3. Nursing—
Planning—Handbooks, manuals, etc.   I. Lederer,
Janet R., 1944-   . [DNLM: 1. Nursing Process—
handbooks.   2. Patient Care Planning—handbooks.
WY 39 C271]
RT49.C37   1986   610.73   85-28797
ISBN 0-201-16305-5

ISBN 0-201-16305-5

DEFGHIJ-AL-8987

Contents

Preface

Y0-CBB-502

The *Care Planning Pocket Guide* is an educational tool designed to help nurses develop the individualized nursing care plans necessary to good patient care. A variety of special features contribute to its usefulness and makes it an indispensable tool for writing care plans.

Features

Organized for easy use   The book is divided into two main parts: (1) complete plans of care, written according to nursing diagnoses, and (2) a list of medical and surgical diagnoses, each accompanied by suggested nursing diagnoses. This unique organization allows you to start with *either* a medical or nursing diagnosis.

Easy to individualize   Each nursing diagnosis has suggested "related to" statements that make it easy to individualize the care plan to the specific patient situation. The authors encourage creativity by suggesting that nurses add specific outcomes, interventions, and "related to" statements in order to tailor the care plan to the individual patient.

Comprehensive   Each plan of care is comprehensive and allows nurses to select specific content according to the patient's condition and situation. Each plan includes (1) "related to" statements, (2) a definition of the nursing diagnosis, (3) subjective and objective defining characteristics, (4) expected outcomes, (5) a reminder to specify the frequency of documentation and expected date of completion, and (6) a list, organized in the steps of the nursing process, of appropriate nursing interventions.

Nursing diagnosis

Nursing diagnoses and care planning help the nurse assess the patient in a holistic way. By defining and organizing knowledge as a basis for practice, and by providing a method of communicating this knowledge among care givers in a systematic way, nursing diagnoses and nursing care plans contribute significantly to the practice of nursing. Nursing diagnoses provide a common language, encourage accountability, and help to define nursing practice as different from medicine.

Nursing diagnoses are a nursing responsibility. They help to provide goals for excellence in patient care. The list of nursing diagnoses used in this book is taken from the most current list published by the North American Nursing Diagnosis Association (NANDA). The diagnoses selected for this book are generic to patients in an acute care setting, with disorders generally defined as medical-surgical.

Audience

This handbook was developed to facilitate care planning. It is equally helpful to nursing students, staff nurses in a variety of clinical settings, and instructors in inservice education settings.

The novice care planner, or the experienced nurse less familiar with nursing diagnoses, may find it helpful to use the list of medical and surgical conditions first. Once the appropriate nursing diagnoses have been selected from this list, the nurse can use the plans of care to formulate individualized, patient-centered care plans. The nurse who is more familiar with the care planning process will find the content in both sections useful in formulating new, creative ways to plan care. The expert in nursing care plans will be able to use this book to extract information that further expresses the needs of the patient and/or family.

Acknowledgments

A special thank you is due to the El Camino Hospital nurses who, as members of the Nurse Care Planning Committee, created the initial care plans that have been used at El Camino Hospital since 1982. These care plans were the basis for the work done on this book.

How to Use This Book

This book has been organized to help nurses prepare individualized care plans. Most of the necessary information is found in "Plans of Care" and in "Nursing Diagnosis Guide to Medical and Surgical Conditions," the two main parts of this book. If the nursing diagnosis for a patient is already established, the nurse can look up that diagnosis in "Plans of Care" before developing the care plan. The nursing diagnoses are organized alphabetically for easy reference.

If the reader is unsure of the appropriate nursing diagnosis for a patient, then the diagnosis guide will assist in that determination. The diagnosis guide lists medical and surgical conditions. Listed under each condition are suggested nursing diagnoses and "related to" statements. After determining the nursing diagnoses, the reader can use "Plans of Care" to review the plans specific to those diagnoses. More specific information regarding these two parts of this book, with some examples of how to use them, follow.

Plans of care

Each plan in this part includes a nursing diagnostic statement (with its definition), defining characteristics, "related to" statements, measurable outcome statements, documentation intervals and target dates, and nursing interventions. Each of these components is introduced briefly under the following headings.

Nursing diagnosis

Each nursing diagnosis should be considered either as a real or a potential problem for the patient and/or family. Most definitions include the words "a condition in which the individual experiences, or could experience . . ." to indicate the reality or potentiality of the nursing diagnosis. Often, it is important to anticipate potential problems that could possibly be prevented by nursing interventions. Although only a few nursing diagnostic categories are officially labeled as "potential," the philosophy of this book is that any nursing diagnosis can be considered potential. When choosing the outcomes and interventions for a potential occurrence, the nurse should be selective, considering those nursing interventions that could prevent the occurrence of a potential problem.

"Related to" statements
■──

The "related to" portion of the diagnostic statement implies a link or connection to the nursing diagnosis but does not necessarily connote a cause-and-effect relationship. The more specific the "related to" statement is, the more specifically the interventions and outcomes can be stated. These specifics help the nurse delineate the appropriate nursing diagnosis. The "related to" statement is not the cause of the nursing diagnosis; rather, it is the reason the nursing diagnosis is appropriate.

Definition
■──

Used in conjunction with the defining characteristics, the definition of each problem found at the beginning of the plan of care helps the nurse verify a particular nursing diagnosis. The definition refers to an observed patient problem that nurses can identify and that warrants nursing intervention. The definition is *not* the medical diagnosis assigned to that patient; it is the *nursing* diagnosis, which responds to nursing measures.

Defining characteristics
■──

Defining characteristics are descriptors of patient behavior, either observed by the nurse or verbalized by the patient. Frequently discovered during the initial nursing history and assessment, the defining characteristics are organized into meaningful groups or patterns of information that alert the nurse to the possibility of an existing patient problem. Usually, the presence of one or two defining characteristics is enough to verify a nursing diagnosis. Occasionally the same descriptors apply to several nursing diagnoses. For example, pallor, shortness of breath, and expressions of anxiety are defining characteristics of many nursing diagnoses. Several descriptors may be used to assess the total picture of the patient and to pinpoint the pertinent nursing diagnosis.

Subjective and objective descriptors are equally important in the validation of a nursing diagnosis. Subjective data originate with the patient; these are data the patient perceives as true. These descriptors are not usually perceived by others. Subjective data include expressions by the patient and family of emotions and physical sensations. Objective data are observable behaviors, characteristics, and information perceived by others. Objective data include nonverbal expressions by the patient and the patient's family or friends. Additionally, objective data include physical assessment data and chart information, such as laboratory values, radiology reports, physician progress notes, nurse's notes, the history and physical, and charting done by ancillary personnel. Both subjective and objective information are necessary considerations during the assessment phase of the nursing process. Both help the nurse to select the appropriate nursing diagnosis.

For example, the patient may state, "I'm having pain in my stomach." The nurse's direct observation produces the following collection of information: "Patient is restless, holds stomach, and refuses breakfast tray with facial grimace." Additionally, the nurse may observe: "Blood pressure elevated to 150/90 mm Hg with pulse rate of 120 beats per minute." The collection of information probably suggests the nursing diagnosis, *Comfort, Alteration in; related to acute pain.* Nurses often confirm the presence of the defining characteristics with the patient to avoid making assumptions or inferences about the characteristics or the problem. When addressing the problem, nurses can frequently include patients in the planning of care.

Outcomes

Outcomes are statements of patient/family behaviors that are measurable, observable, and denote a desired goal. Outcome statements, like all components of the care planning process, are dynamic. Outcomes, therefore, are frequently changing goals. Some goals are easily achieved and, once accomplished, can be deleted. Others may take longer to achieve and need periodic reevaluation. Measurable outcome statements are critical. Without them, the care planning process has no evaluation component.

Not all outcomes listed will be appropriate for each patient. To determine the relevant outcome, the nurse consults the initial assessment data; the outcome will change as patient behavior changes. Partial behavior change may be the most realistic goal, since length of stay varies depending upon hospital service and geographic region. The patient goal may need to be completed after discharge, by supervised health professionals in the community setting. Discussion with the patient may be initiated to determine patient/family goals still needing completion.

The nurse should select outcome statements carefully for attainability because the evaluation portion of the care plan measures whether or not the goal is met. For this reason, the nurse may need to write an outcome statement that is specific to the patient/family situation in addition to using one in this handbook. More than one outcome statement may be necessary.

The evaluation process is incomplete unless a documentation interval and a target date accompany the outcome statement. These three components are reviewed for currency and applicability at least daily and changed as the patient's condition or situation changes.

Documentation interval

The documentation interval designates when patient behaviors should be documented. Because it is important to specify the frequency of documentation, each plan of care reminds the nurse to specify the documentation interval. This interval should be determined during initial assessment and may change as patient behaviors indicate the completion of a goal. For example, the outcome "Vital signs will be within normal limits for patient" is documented when vital signs are taken. The documentation interval could be specified as the anticipated frequency of occurrence, such as q2 hours, q8 hours, qid, or q2 days.

Target date

The target date is the estimated date a goal will be met. The date is individualized to the patient, is flexible, and should be reviewed periodically. Each care plan reminds the reader to specify an expected target date. A specific target date is selected to encourage documentation that is specific and that indicates whether the desired outcome is being achieved. Target dates are changed as necessary. The target date, and its subsequent review, help the nurse document the patient outcomes.

Interventions

The interventions listed for each plan of care include activities performed throughout the nursing process: assessment, planning, interventions, and evaluation. The interventions are grouped according to the steps of the nursing process and should be chosen only if they apply to the patient's condition and circumstance. For example, it may be necessary to select only a few of the interventions at first and add others later as necessary. The nurse may need to write interventions specifically for an individualized care plan. In certain instances, "q ____" is included in the intervention statement to remind the nurse to individualize the intervention. In other words, the nurse must intervene as often as the nature of the task requires and in accordance with the patient's condition.

Often, assessment and documentation information is included in an intervention statement. Documentation is essential to quantify nursing actions. This documentation should include the type of nursing intervention, its frequency, and the patient's response. Without this documentation, the patient's progress cannot be evaluated.

Certain interventions require assessment of laboratory values available in the patient's chart. Normal ranges for laboratory values vary with the clinical laboratory equipment used in different facilities, and the nurse may need to refer to other resources to evaluate the patient's laboratory results.

In addition to using the interventions listed in the handbook, the nurse needs to add interventions that are specific to the patient's situation. This step ensures that the care plan is individualized. As the patient's condition changes, interventions may be added, changed, or deleted. Frequent updating of this portion of the care plan is essential.

Nursing process and development of plans of care

The nursing process is put to use continuously during the rendering of nursing care in every clinical setting. Many components of the nursing process overlap and often are repeated, making all aspects of nursing care dynamic. It is important to consider the patient as the central figure in the plan of care. The nurse must confirm appropriateness of all aspects of nursing care by observing the patient's response to the treatment, be it medical, surgical, or psychosocial.

Figure 1 displays the relationships among the steps in the nursing process and the components of the individualized plan of care.

The assessment portion of the nursing process is the collection of data derived from patient observation and from the patient's clinical response to treatment. The appropriate nursing diagnosis is determined at this time. The definition and defining characteristics help the nurse in this process. Once the nursing diagnosis is determined, the plan of care is created. To do so, the nurse uses the planning portion of the nursing process and decides on the outcome statements and needed interventions. Implementing the interventions is the next task. After implementation, the nurse assesses, plans, and evaluates the appropriateness of

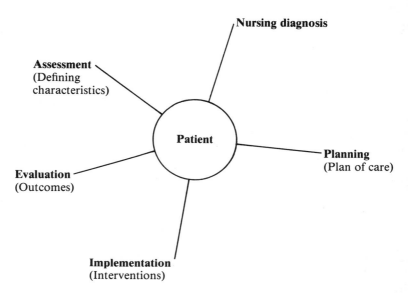

Figure 1. Interactions among steps of nursing process and components of care plans.

the plan of care continuously. The outcome statements are the evaluation portion of the plan of care. As such, they must be measurable. The nurse evaluates patient behaviors to determine whether outcomes are completed or partially completed. The documentation interval and target date help the nurse project the completion of the outcome.

All components of the plan of care are important. The plan of care is incomplete without a continuous determination of the appropriateness of each component.

Nursing diagnoses guide to medical and surgical conditions

The second main part of this handbook is set up to help the nurse select nursing diagnoses when the patient's medical diagnosis is known but the appropriate nursing diagnoses have not yet been established. In this section, medical and surgical conditions are listed, along with related nursing diagnoses and "related to" statements. When reviewing these lists, the nurse needs to remember that not all of the nursing diagnoses will apply to each patient situation. He or she should select only those nursing diagnoses that are determined to be applicable from the assessment information collected. Once a nursing diagnosis is selected, the "related to" statement is chosen. It may be necessary to write a "related to" statement that is specific to the patient's situation rather than using one that is already listed. The nurse needs to keep in mind that the "related to" statement is not the cause of the nursing diagnosis; rather, it is the reason the nursing diagnosis is appropriate.

The list of medical and surgical conditions does not include rare disease conditions, and it may be necessary to refer to a more general title. For example, the patient's medical diagnosis may be poliomyelitis. Since this condition occurs rarely, the nurse should look under the general title *Immobilized patient* and review the nursing diagnoses listed there before developing the care plan.

After selecting the nursing diagnoses, the reader can refer to "Plans of Care."

Case example

The following example shows how to use this book to create a care plan in a specific situation. It illustrates the application of nursing process in the selection of a nursing diagnosis and the subsequent development of a plan of care.

Mr. A, a 25-year-old male, has been admitted to a surgical unit from the emergency department with the medical diagnosis of appendicitis. He has been scheduled for an emergency appendectomy. On admission, he complains of nausea and right lower quadrant pain, which became noticeable while he was working at his office. He moans, grimaces, and splints his abdomen with his arms. He asks for pain medication. He is unmarried, employed as an engineer, and lives alone. This is his first hospitalization. He is taking no medications and has no known allergies. He states that he is nervous about being in the hospital. He asks when he will be able to return to work and resume his normal activity.

Mr. A's admission medical orders include:

Start an intravenous solution

NPO except for ice

Monitor intake and output

Give intramuscular pain medication

Administer antibiotic via piggyback IV line

Take vital signs qid

7

Ambulate, as tolerated

CBC and urinalysis

Your assessment of Mr. A reveals the following information. His vital signs are: blood pressure 118/70 mm Hg, radial pulse rate 100 beats per minute and regular, respirations 28 breaths per minute, and temperature 100.0 F orally. Abdominal assessment reveals bowel sounds in all quadrants and pain in the right lower quadrant on palpation, with distinct rebound tenderness. Laboratory results show the CBC to be normal, except for the WBC count elevation to 13,000. Urinalysis results are normal.

The admission data have been collected, and it is now time to determine the appropriate nursing diagnoses and plans of care for Mr. A. The following process can be used in this determination.

Mr. A has complained of nausea and pain and is requesting pain medication. His pulse rate and respiratory rate are both higher than normal. He is holding his abdomen trying to splint the painful area. It is probable that one applicable nursing diagnosis is *Comfort, Alteration in*. All of the assessment data match these descriptors. The choice of this nursing diagnosis is appropriate for Mr. A.

If the nurse is unsure which nursing diagnoses are appropriate for Mr. A, or if the nurse wants to review additional possible nursing diagnoses, he or she refers to page 136 to look over the list of nursing diagnoses appropriate for *Abdominal surgery* (including appendectomy). The nurse then uses the assessment data to determine which of the listed nursing diagnoses is appropriate for Mr. A's care plan.

Now it is time to determine the measurable outcomes. Two outcomes that could be selected are:

Patient reports absence of or decrease in pain.

Patient requests pain medication.

Both outcomes are measurable and appropriate. The documentation interval for each would be every 8 hours, and the target date would be 2 to 3 days from admission and surgery. The nurse should give a real date as the target date. The documentation interval and target date should be reviewed at least daily to ensure their appropriateness. The outcome statements are the evaluation portion of the care plan. Mr. A will either verbalize absence of pain, or he won't. He will verbalize the need for pain medication, or he won't. In either case, both of these statements are important as an evaluation portion of the nurse's interaction with Mr. A.

At this point, the nursing interventions are selected. The following interventions may be selected for Mr. A's plan of care:

Ask patient to rate pain on a scale of 0–10 (0 = no pain; 10 = worst pain). Document intensity of pain in nurse's notes.

Explain reason for pain medication and instruct patient to ask for pain medication before pain becomes too severe, as needed.

Be alert to nonverbal cues regarding level of pain.

Offer position change, back rubs, transcutaneous electrical nerve stimulation (TENS), and relaxation techniques as supplements/alternatives to medication for pain relief, depending on the identified level and intensity of pain. Help patient identify measures that have worked in the past.

Maintain therapeutic blood level of medications to ensure optimal pain relief by titration of pain medications.

Help patient focus on activities rather than on pain by providing diversion through television, radio, tapes, and visitors.

Inform patient of procedures that may increase pain.

Encourage patient to request additional pain medication in preparation for procedures that may increase pain.

All of the aforementioned interventions should be part of Mr. A's care. This will ensure consistency in the care provided. Once an intervention is no longer applicable, it should be deleted from the care plan.

Depending on the assessment data, other nursing diagnoses could be applicable in a case study such as this one. This illustration shows the process used to develop a care plan through nursing diagnostic statements, outcome, documentation, target date, and interventions. Figure 2 relates this care plan to the steps of the nursing process.

Nursing process and nursing diagnosis

Care planning is essential to nursing practice. Using the nursing process to create a plan of care provides a structure for nursing practice. A written plan of care ensures that the patient receives physical, social, psychological, and humanistic care that takes into account the patient's needs. Care planning allows the nurse to express creativity in the continued assessment and development of plans of care that are individualized to the patient. Care planning is a communication tool between nurses and other health care providers; this communication ensures continuity of care for each patient.

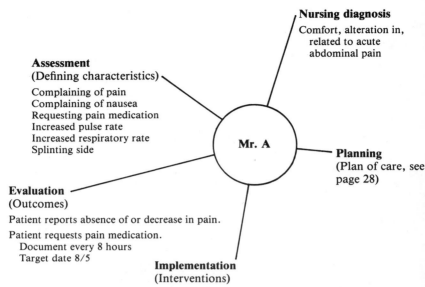

Nursing diagnosis
Comfort, alteration in, related to acute abdominal pain

Assessment
(Defining characteristics)

Complaining of pain
Complaining of nausea
Requesting pain medication
Increased pulse rate
Increased respiratory rate
Splinting side

Mr. A

Planning
(Plan of care, see page 28)

Evaluation
(Outcomes)

Patient reports absence of or decrease in pain.

Patient requests pain medication.
Document every 8 hours
Target date 8/5

Implementation
(Interventions)

Ask patient to rate pain on a scale of 0–10 (0 = no pain; 10 = worst pain). Document intensity of pain in nurse's notes.

Explain reason for pain medication and instruct patient to ask for pain medication before pain becomes too severe, as needed.

Be alert to nonverbal cues regarding level of pain.

Offer position change, back rubs, transcutaneous electrical nerve stimulation (TENS), and relaxation techniques as supplements/alternatives to medication for pain relief, depending on the identified level and intensity of pain. Help patient identify measures that have worked in the past.

Maintain therapeutic blood level of medications to ensure optimal pain relief by titration of pain medications.

Help patient focus on activities rather than on pain by providing diversion through television, radio, tapes, and visitors.

Inform patient of procedures that may increase pain.

Encourage patient to request additional pain medication in preparation for procedures that may increase pain.

Figure 2. Interactions among steps of nursing process and components of care plans for Mr. A.

Patient problems are best viewed from the perspective of the nursing process. What process is used to determine the appropriate diagnostic statement for the patient? Assessment and data collection are imperative as the initial steps in determining which nursing diagnoses apply. The nurse compares the initial assessment data to the descriptors in order to choose the appropriate nursing diagnosis.

To plan for patient care, the nurse selects the relevant outcome statement, including the patient's perceptions and suggestions for the outcome, if possible. Only those outcomes that are specific to the patient are selected. Not all outcomes apply to every situation.

The nurse correlates the nursing interventions with the implementation phase of the nursing process, taking into consideration the fact that this phase of patient care is a dynamic. It is necessary to choose those interventions that are specific to the etiology of the problem and to provide assistance that will return the patient to optimal health.

Evaluation is part of the entire care planning process. This is a continuous series of actions to maintain a current and relevant plan of care for the patient. Evaluation information includes observation of patient behavior as well as documentation. Has the patient reached the outcome chosen for him or her initially? Are certain interventions no longer needed? As evaluation reveals whether the outcome statements have been achieved, the nurse is lead back to the assessment process and the reevaluation of the diagnostic statement.

The use of nursing diagnosis with plans of care provides a link to the standards of care so necessary in health care facilities. Standards of care are the criteria used to gauge both proficiency in the performance of a job and the quality of that performance. The development of a care plan in the context of the nursing process and the documentation of the care provided assist in the development of these standards. Additionally, these components quantify the adherence to the standards. Standards of care are developed for use by all clinical services and should be updated as nursing practice indicates. The use of nursing diagnosis and plans of care provides data for this dynamic process.

Nursing diagnosis development

Since 1973, NANDA members have collaborated in the development of a list of diagnostic statements. The most current accepted list was established in 1982, and input and suggestions from practicing nurses, as well as clinical research submitted to NANDA, are expected to refine the accepted list further. This 1982 list has been used in the development of the plans of care and the nursing diagnosis guides included in this book.

A common language for practicing nurses has long been needed. As nurses use the nursing diagnosis list, they will influence many aspects of patient care in their professional practice. Communication with other health care professionals will be enhanced, ensuring comprehensive and consistent patient care from nurse to nurse, unit to unit, and institution to institution.

The importance of nursing diagnosis in care planning is attested to by many nurses, both in professional literature and clinical practice. The use of nursing diagnosis in care planning formulation certainly makes care planning terminology consistent and universally understandable. Nurses working in various settings, including hospitals, the community, extended care facilities, or occupational health, will benefit from the use of nursing diagnosis.

Health care reimbursement is changing, leading to a shortened hospital stay. Governmental budget restraints and third-party payment reforms will lead to new payment structures. It will be important to quantify patient care for reimbursement. The use of nursing diagnosis and care planning will help the professional nurse to quantify the care given to patients.

No longer are patients remaining in the hospital until they achieve optimal wellness. Discharge is considered appropriate when the patient demonstrates the ability to function somewhat independently or when community resources can be used to help the patient and family gain optimal function. Home care is burgeoning in most communities. Activities once thought appropriate only for the hospital setting are now being done in the home by professional nurses and/or home health aides. It is important that nurses consider this transition from hospital to home or from hospital to skilled nursing facility when they develop and update a plan of care. Continuity in the plans of hospital staff and community staff is very important when patients are discharged. The use of nursing diagnosis and plans of care promotes this continuity. The developed patient care plan can be sent to the community agency when the patient is discharged from the acute care facility.

Plans of Care

Activity intolerance

Related to: Anxiety, Arrhythmias, Impaired gas exchange, Pain (acute or chronic), Weakness/fatigue, Others specific to patient.

A condition in which the individual could experience, or is experiencing, an inability to sustain or increase activity

Defining characteristics

Subjective

Complaining of fatigue
Complaining of feeling faint
Complaining of acute or chronic pain
Complaining of shortness of breath
Complaining of weakness

Objective

Inability to begin activity
Decrease in activity level
Pain
Increased or decreased blood
  pressure
Increased pulse rate/thready pulse
Irregular pulse
Increased respiratory rate
Rapid, shallow respirations
Diaphoresis
Pallor

Outcomes

Patient identifies activities that increase fatigue.

Patient verbalizes importance of pacing activities with appropriate rest periods.

Patient identifies anxiety-producing situations that may contribute to activity intolerance.

Patient demonstrates ability to intersperse activity with appropriate rest periods.

Patient verbalizes understanding of need to participate in required physical activity.

Patient demonstrates ability to perform activities with increased comfort.

Patient employs safety measures to minimize potential for injury.

Patient verbalizes understanding of need for equipment, such as oxygen, that increases tolerance for activities.

Other outcomes specific to patient (specify).

Documentation

Specify frequency.

Target date

Specify estimated date of completion.

Nursing interventions
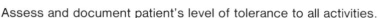

Assess and document patient's level of tolerance to all activities.

Assess and document presence of arrhythmia, shortness of breath, dizziness, pain, and diaphoresis as indicators of limited tolerance for activity.

Encourage patient to report onset of pain, including severity, location, and precipitating activities. Document in nurse's notes.

Encourage patient to request pain medication prior to beginning activity, as necessary.

Encourage patient to verbalize activities that increase fatigue.

Instruct patient in use of equipment, such as oxygen, that facilitates activity and in the use of relaxation techniques during activities.

Instruct patient in ways to identify and decrease anxiety-producing situations.

Plan activities with patient/family that minimize fatigue.

Set small, realistic, attainable goals with patient that increase independence and self-esteem.

Provide rest periods between and during activities.

Promote independence in activity within energy limits of patient.

Contract with patient regarding increase in activity. Document plan in nurse's notes.

Provide positive reinforcement for increased activity.

Assist with activity, as needed.

Provide safe environment by removing obstacles from ambulation area.

Keep frequently used objects within easy reach of patient.

Include family in assisting with activities, as appropriate.

Other interventions specific to patient (specify).

Anxiety

Related to: Specific to patient.

A condition in which the individual experiences, or could experience, vague feelings of uneasiness that threaten the individual's self-worth and self-esteem

Defining characteristics

Subjective

Verbalizing increased tension
Expressing insecurity
Verbalizing unfocused apprehension
Verbalizing helplessness
Expressing stress
Expressing ambivalence
Verbalizing unmet expectations
Verbalizing a lack of control
Verbalizing an anticipated change in life situation
Verbalizing feelings of regret
Focusing on past events

Objective

Irritability
Restlessness
Increased pulse rate
Poor eye contact
High-pitched voice
Trembling
Perspiration
Facial flushing
Crying
Wringing of hands
Shuffling of feet
Hand tremors
Urinary frequency
Increased gastrointestinal activity
Change in eating habits
Inability to learn
Insomnia

Outcomes

Patient verbalizes anxiety.

Patient verbalizes events that precipitate anxiety.

Patient verbalizes reduction in anxiety.

Patient verbalizes increased awareness of environment.

Patient verbalizes techniques that reduce anxiety.

Patient demonstrates ability to use techniques that have reduced anxiety in the past.

Patient demonstrates ability to continue with necessary activities even though anxiety persists.

Patient verbalizes a decrease in somatic complaints.

Patient demonstrates ability to retain knowledge and skills.

Other outcomes specific to patient (specify).

Documentation

■──

Specify frequency.

Target date

■──

Specify estimated date of completion.

Nursing interventions

■──

Assess and document presence of anxiety by observing the patient's behavior.

Assess and document patient's unmet needs and expectations by encouraging patient to express thoughts and feelings.

Help patient identify events that have precipitated anxiety in the past.

Explore with patient techniques that have, and have not, reduced anxiety in the past.

Help patient focus on the present situation as a means of identifying coping mechanisms needed to reduce anxiety.

Reassure patient during interactions by touch and empathetic verbal and nonverbal exchanges, encourage patient to express anger and irritation, and allow patient to cry.

Reduce excess stimulation by providing a quiet environment, limited contact with others if necessary, and limited use of caffeine and other stimulants.

Suggest alternative methods of reducing anxiety that are acceptable to patient.

Provide diversion through television, radio, games, and occupational therapies to reduce anxiety and expand focus.

Provide positive reinforcement when patient is able to continue with activities of daily living and other activities necessary to progress to optimal wellness.

Develop teaching plan with realistic goals including need for repetition, encouragement, and praise of the tasks learned.

Other interventions specific to patient (specify).

■──

Bowel elimination, Alteration in:
Constipation

Related to: Aging process, Decreased activity, Decreased fluid intake, Dietary changes, Disease process, Medications (specify), Painful defecation, Others specific to patient.

An individual's episodic condition in which feces are, or could be, infrequent, dry, or hard, in contrast to the individual's normal pattern

Defining characteristics

Subjective

Changing bowel pattern
Changing lifestyle
Complaining of decreased appetite
Complaining of indigestion
Complaining of painful defecation/ cramping
Complaining of rectal fullness, abdominal fullness, or pain
Complaining of straining upon defecating

Objective

Absence of bowel sounds
Increase or decrease in bowel sounds
Distended abdomen
Passage of liquid/loose stool
Hard, formed stool
Perianal redness of skin

Outcomes

Patient is free of abdominal distention.

Patient has bowel sounds on auscultation.

Patient verbalizes the passage of flatus.

Patient verbalizes presence of optimal bowel pattern.

Patient passes stool of usual consistency for patient.

Patient shows knowledge by describing dietary requirements to maintain usual bowel pattern.

Patient is free of skin irritation, perianal redness, and hard stool.

Patient verbalizes the passage of stool with a reduction in pain.

Patient verbalizes the passage of stool without straining.

Patient demonstrates knowledge of bowel regimen necessary to overcome the side-effects of medications.

Other outcomes specific to patient (specify).

Documentation
■──

Specify frequency.

Target date
■──

Specify estimated date of completion.

Nursing interventions
■──

Assess and document presence or absence of bowel sounds in all
     four quadrants q ____.
Assess and document abdominal distention by palpating abdomen in all
     four quadrants q ____.
Document the passage of flatus.
Assess and document impaction q ____.
Assess and document condition of perianal skin q ____.
Request the patient to identify his or her usual bowel pattern to gather
     baseline data on bowel regimen, activity, and medications. Docu-
     ment usual pattern in nurse's notes.
Encourage patient to request pain medication prior to defecation in
     order to facilitate painless passage of stool.
Document the color and consistency of first stool postoperatively.
Document frequency, color, and consistency of stool.
Encourage optimal activity to stimulate patient's bowel activity.
Provide fluids of patient's choice (specify).
Consult with dietitian for increased fiber in diet.
Request a physician's order for elimination aids, such as dietary bran,
     stool softeners, and laxatives.
Stress the avoidance of straining when defecating to prevent change in
     vital signs, dizziness, or bleeding.
Provide privacy and safety for patient during bowel elimination.
Provide care in an accepting, nonjudgmental manner.
Inform patient of possibility of medication-induced constipation.
Instruct patient in bowel elimination aids that promote optimal bowel
     pattern at home.
Other interventions specific to patient (specify).

■──

Bowel elimination, Alteration in: *Diarrhea*

Related to: Dietary changes, Disease process (specify), Impaction, Medications (specify), Stress, Others specific to patient.

An individual's episodic condition in which feces are, or could be, frequent, loose, or fluid, in contrast with the individual's normal pattern

Defining characteristics

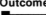

Subjective

Complaining of abdominal cramping
Complaining of abdominal pain
Complaining of urgency to defecate
Complaining of decreased appetite

Objective

Change in usual consistency, frequency, and volume of stool
Involuntary stool
Loose/liquid stool
Weight loss
Fluid and electrolyte imbalances

Outcomes

Patient verbalizes presence of optimal bowel pattern.

Patient passes stool of usual consistency.

Patient verbalizes the stressors that may contribute to diarrhea.

Patient passes stool with decreasing frequency.

Patient shows knowledge by describing dietary requirements to maintain usual bowel pattern.

Patient has weight gain.

Other outcomes specific to patient (specify).

Documentation
■────────────────────────────────────

Specify frequency.

Target date
■────────────────────────────────────

Specify estimated date of completion.

Nursing interventions
■────────────────────────────────────

Assess and document frequency, color, and consistency of stool.

Assess and document impaction q ＿＿.

Assess and document condition of perianal skin q ＿＿.

Assess and document evidence of electrolyte imbalances.

Assess and document skin turgor and condition of oral mucosa as indicators of dehydration.

Weigh patient daily, as indicated.

Assess for malnutrition and vitamin deficiencies that may be induced by weight and fluid loss.

Assess and document urinary output as an indicator of dehydration.

Request patient to identify patient's usual bowel pattern. Document usual pattern in nurse's notes.

Encourage patient to identify stressors that may contribute to diarrhea.

Document in nurse's notes the patient's assessment of stressors.

Request physician's order for antidiarrhetic, antispasmotic medications.

Inform patient of possibility of medication-induced diarrhea.

Provide care in an accepting, nonjudgmental manner.

Provide fluids of patient's choice (specify).

Consult with dietitian for increased fiber in diet.

Stress the avoidance of straining when defecating.

Provide privacy and safety for patient during bowel elimination.

Instruct patient in diet and use of antidiarrhetic medications to promote optimal bowel pattern at home.

Other interventions specific to patient (specify).

■────────────────────────────────────

Bowel elimination, Alteration in:
Incontinence

■━━━━━━━━━━━━━━━━━━━━━━━━━━━━━━━━━━━

Related to: Decreased awareness of need to defecate, Disease process (specify), Loss of sphincter control, Others specific to patient.

A condition in which an individual experiences, or could experience, involuntary evacuation of fecal material

Defining characteristics
■━━━━━━━━━━━━━━━━━━━━━━━━━━━━━━━━━━━

Subjective

Complaining of involuntary stool
Complaining of urgency

Objective

Liquid stool
Formed stool
Reddened perianal skin

Outcomes
■━━━━━━━━━━━━━━━━━━━━━━━━━━━━━━━━━━━

Patient is not incontinent.

Patient verbalizes presence of optimal bowel pattern.

Patient passes stool of usual consistency for patient.

Patient shows knowledge by describing dietary requirements to maintain usual bowel pattern.

Patient is free of skin irritation of perianal area.

Other outcomes specific to patient (specify).

Documentation
■───

Specify frequency.

Target date
■───

Specify estimated date of completion.

Nursing interventions
■───

Assess and document frequency, color, and consistency of stool.

Assess and document for bowel impaction q ＿＿.

Assess and document condition of perianal skin after each episode of incontinence. Document condition of perianal skin q ＿＿.

Request patient to identify own bowel pattern. Document usual pattern in nurse's notes.

Provide clothing to protect patient's skin from involuntary stool.

Provide bedpan or assist to commode q ＿＿.

Institute bowel training program. Specify bowel training program appropriate for patient.

Document bowel routine specific to patient.

Provide care in an accepting, nonjudgmental manner.

Request physician's order for medications that decrease episodes of incontinence.

Provide fluids of patients' choice (specify).

Consult with dietitian for increased fiber in diet.

Provide privacy and safety for patient.

Other interventions specific to patient (specify).

■───

Cardiac output, Alteration in: *Decreased*

■━━━━━━━━━━━━━━━━━━━━━

Related to: Arrhythmia, Drug intolerance, Drug side-effects, Stress on heart's function, Others specific to patient.

A condition in which an individual experiences, or could experience, a decrease in output of blood from the heart resulting in accumulation and/or displacement of circulating blood volume

Defining characteristics
■━━━━━━━━━━━━━━━━━━━━━

Subjective

Complaining of chest pain
Complaining of dizziness
Complaining of fatigue
Complaining of listlessness
Complaining of weakness
Expressing difficulty in breathing

Objective

Agitation
Dyspnea
Decreased circulation to extremities
Cyanosis
Decreased level of consciousness
Dependent edema
Diaphoresis
Distended neck veins
Increased or decreased pulse rate
Low blood pressure/orthostatic
    hypotension
Moist rales
Urinary output less than 30cc/hour
Seizures

Outcomes
■━━━━━━━━━━━━━━━━━━━━━

Patient maintains regular apical pulse.

Patient maintains irregular, non—life threatening apical rhythm.

Patient maintains sinus rhythm, or controlled atrial fibrillation on monitored patient.

Patient verbalizes onset, duration, and precipitating factors of chest pain.

Patient's vital signs are within normal limits for patient. Specify normal limits for pressure, pulse, and respirations.

Patient has decreased peripheral edema.

Outcomes *(continued)*

Patient verbalizes fewer subjective symptoms.
Patient verbalizes understanding of medications.
Patient's urinary output is greater than 30cc/hour.
Other outcomes specific to patient (specify).

Documentation

Specify frequency.

Target date

Specify estimated date of completion.

Nursing interventions

Auscultate and document the quality of the apical pulse q ____.
Correlate baseline vital signs with current vital signs to assess for any changes in blood pressure; pulse (rate, rhythm, quality); and respirations.
Assess and document effects of O_2 on arrhythmias correlating presence and/or absence of arrhythmias.
Assess and document effects of antiarrhythmic medications on arrhythmias.
Assess and document effects of other cardiac and noncardiac medications on heart function.
Assess and document presence of peripheral edema as indicators of fluid retention.
Assess and document effects of anxiety/stress on arrhythmias.
Instruct patient to report onset, duration, and precipitating factors of palpitations, chest pain, or shortness of breath.
Instruct patient to notify nurse of pain including site, quality, intensity, duration, and precipitating events.
Auscultate lungs for adventitious sounds as indicators of fluid overload. Document in nurse's notes.
Assess and document intake and output. Maintain urinary output at 30cc/hour, noting color, amount, and consistency.

(continued)

Nursing interventions *(continued)*

Assess and document patient's tolerance to activity by noting onset of shortness of breath, chest pain, palpitations, or dizziness.

Correlate and document increase in activity level with presence of arrhythmias.

Increase patient's activity level to patient's tolerance.

Change patient's position to flat/Trendelenberg when blood pressure is in lower than normal range for patient. Document patient's response to position change.

Correlate patient's blood pressure with blood pressure medications administered. Withhold blood pressure medications when there is a drop in blood pressure and notify physician.

For prolonged hypotension, establish intravenous access for administration of intravenous fluids and/or medications to raise blood pressure.

Correlate and document rhythm with laboratory values, vital signs, peripheral perfusions, and/or effects of treatment.

Explain purpose and function of cardiac monitor to patient.

Maintain adequate oxygenation by administering O_2 per nasal cannula or mask.

Instruct patient on medications, including name, dose, frequency, and potential side-effects. Document instruction in nurse's notes.

Provide home instruction to patient and family on activity limitations, use of therapeutic equipment, and signs and symptoms that may require notification of physician.

Other interventions specific to patient (specify).

■——————————————————————————————

Comfort, Alteration in

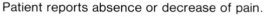

Related to: Bed rest, Pain (acute), Others specific to patient. (See also following diagnosis.)

An episodic condition in which the individual experiences, or could experience, verbal or nonverbal indicators of physical, emotional, or psychological discomfort

Defining characteristics

Subjective

Complaining of pain, discomfort
Complaining of nausea
Requesting medication for pain relief

Objective

Increased blood pressure
Increased/decreased pulse rate
Increased respiratory rate
Pallor, diaphoresis
Limited movement, slow movement
Splinting incision or other pain site
Crying
Flat affect
Grimacing
Restlessness
Limited attention span
Withdrawal

Outcomes

Patient reports absence or decrease of pain.

Patient verbalizes reasonable comfort.

Patient requests pain/comfort medications.

Patient demonstrates individualized relaxation techniques that are effective for pain control.

Other outcomes specific to patient (specify).

Documentation

Specify frequency.

Target date

Specify estimated date of completion.

Nursing interventions
■————————————————————————————————————

Convey to patient that assessment of pain entails understanding patient's perception of pain, not determining the presence or absence of pain.

Ask patient to rate pain on a scale of 0–10 (0 = no pain; 10 = worst pain). Document intensity of pain in nurse's notes.

Explain reason for pain medication and instruct patient to ask for pain medication before pain becomes too severe, as needed.

Be alert to pain behaviors related to religion, culture, and beliefs that may influence the patient's perception of pain.

Be alert to nonverbal cues regarding level of pain.

Offer position change, back rubs, transcutaneous electrical nerve stimulation (TENS), and relaxation techniques as supplements/alternatives to medication for pain relief, depending on the identified level and intensity of pain. Help patient identify measures that have worked in the past.

Administer pain medications prior to activities/procedures.

Maintain therapeutic blood level of medications to ensure optimal pain relief by titration of pain medications.

Assess and document patient's response to pain management without projecting the nurse's own values and beliefs about pain.

Encourage patient to maintain optimal activity level.

Provide care in an unhurried, supportive manner.

Involve patient in decisions regarding care activities.

Help patient focus on activities rather than on pain by providing diversion through television, radio, tapes, and visitors.

Confer with physician on pain management and assess need for change in pain medication order, as needed.

Discuss with patient/family pain management regimen to provide maximal comfort.

Inform patient of procedures that may increase pain.

Encourage patient to request additional pain medication in preparation for procedures that may increase pain.

Other interventions specific to patient (specify).

■————————————————————————————————————

Comfort, Alteration in

■

Related to: Pain (chronic), Others specific to patient. (See also preceding diagnosis.)

A condition in which the individual experiences, or could experience, verbal or nonverbal indicators of physical, emotional, or psychological discomfort that has existed over time

Defining characteristics
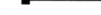

Subjective

Complaining of pain, discomfort
Requesting medication for pain relief
Complaining of frustration
Complaining of depression
Complaining of nausea

Objective

Crying
Flat affect
Grimacing
Anorexia
Fatigue
Limited movement
Slow movements
Limited attention span
Insomnia
Withdrawal

Outcomes
■

Patient reports reasonable comfort.

Patient verbalizes increasing ability to cope with pain.

Patient demonstrates knowledge of adaptive measures for pain relief.

Patient demonstrates ability to tolerate pain.

Other outcomes specific to patient (specify).

Documentation
■

Specify frequency.

Target date
■

Specify estimated date of completion.

Nursing interventions
■

Identify and document situations that may potentiate pain.

Identify and document techniques that reduce pain.

Convey to patient that assessment of pain entails understanding the patient's perception of pain, not determining the presence or absence of pain.

Encourate patient to identify previously effective coping mechanisms for pain. Document in nurse's notes.

Ask patient to rate pain on a scale of 0–10 (0 = no pain; 10 = worst pain). Document patient's perception of pain intensity.

Assess and document effects of long-term medication use.

Be alert to verbal and nonverbal cues regarding level of pain experienced by patient.

Convey to patient that total pain relief may not be achievable.

Encourage patient to inform nurse if pain relief is not achieved.

Establish pain management routine specific to patient. Document routine in nurse's notes.

Encourage patient to maintain optimal activity level.

Pace care activities as appropriate to patient's pain level.

Involve patient in discussions regarding care, incorporating patient's methods of pain relief in care.

Provide care in an unhurried, supportive manner, allowing for sufficient rest periods.

Discuss with patient pain relief measures to supplement pain medication, such as biofeedback, relaxation techniques, back rub, and imagery.

Document patient's response to pain relief measures.

Discuss with patient/family pain management regimen to provide maximal comfort at home.

Other interventions specific to patient (specify).

■

Communication, Impaired: *Verbal*

Related to: Acute confusion, Aphasia (expressive and receptive), Inability to speak, Primary language other than English, Others specific to patient.

A condition in which the individual is unable, or could be unable, to express and/or understand thoughts, feelings, and needs so that they are understood by others

Defining characteristics

Subjective

Complaining of not being understood by others
Lacking ability to follow instructions
Lacking ability to answer questions

Objective

Absence of audible speech
Communication in foreign language
Exaggerated descriptive speech
Garbled, nonsensical speech
Incompletely expressed thoughts
Medical regimen/disease process interfering with audible sounds (i.e., CVA, ET tube, tracheotomy)
Sign language primary mode of communication
Receptive/expressive verbalization deficit
Shortness of breath

Outcomes

Patient communicates needs to staff with minimal frustration.

Patient demonstrates increased ability to express needs to staff and family.

Patient demonstrates understanding of need to change communication system in order to express needs to staff and family.

Patient expresses anger, frustration, sorrow related to inability to communicate needs to staff and family.

Patient demonstrates increased understanding of spoken words and gestures.

Patient communicates satisfaction with alternate means of communication.

Other outcomes specific to patient (specify).

Documentation

Specify frequency.

Target date

Specify estimated date of completion.

Nursing interventions

Assess and document patient's communication pattern to facilitate optimal two-way communication.

Assess and document patient's ability to speak, hear, write, read, and understand in order to establish communication between staff and patient, and family and patient.

Explain to patient why he or she cannot speak, if applicable.

Identify and document patient's primary language.

Encourage self-expression by patient in any manner that provides information to staff/family to ensure that patient's needs are being met.

Utilize flash cards, pad/pencil, gestures, pictures, foreign language vocabulary lists, and the like to facilitate optimal two-way communication.

Encourage patient to communicate slowly and to repeat requests, using alternative methods of communication, if necessary.

Reassure patient that frustration and anger is acceptable and expected.

Encourage frequent visiting by family/significant others to provide stimulation for communication.

Involve the patient and family in development of communication plan.

Speak slowly, distinctly, quietly, facing the patient.

Provide care in a relaxed, unhurried, nonjudgmental manner.

Provide continuity in nursing assignment to establish trust and reduce frustration.

Use nursing care plan to identify established communication system and to ensure continuity of care.

Consult with physician regarding need for speech therapy, if appropriate.

Give frequent positive reinforcement to patient to encourage communication with staff and family.

Use family/significant person as translator, as appropriate.

Be aware of cultural patterns that may influence communication, such as touch, spatial distance when speaking, and role of males/females. Document patterns that may demonstrate cultural influence in the nursing care plan.

Utilize hospital translator, when available.

Other interventions specific to patient (specify).

Coping, Ineffective individual

Related to: Aggression, Anger, Anxiety, Denial, Depression, Others specific to patient. (See also following diagnosis.)

A condition in which an individual could be unable, or is unable, to maintain his or her usual level of functioning in physical, emotional, or psychological support of self because of actual or perceived changes in the environment

Defining characteristics

Subjective

Expressing unrealistic expectations
Expressing anger
Expressing anxiety
Expressing inability to accept situation
Expressing depression
States, "I can't cope."
Complaining of altered eating habits
Complaining of altered elimination patterns
Making exaggerated somatic complaints
Expressing sleep pattern disruption

Objective

Agitation
Manipulative/aggressive behavior
Unwillingness to participate in self-care
Verbal hostility between patient, family, and staff
Withdrawal

Outcomes

Patient verbalizes anger.

Patient verbalizes anxiety.

Patient acknowledges inability to accept situation.

Patient verbalizes depression.

Patient participates in activities of daily living.

Patient demonstrates interest in diversions and recreation.

Patient initiates conversation.

Patient reacts with verbal and nonverbal responses applicable to situation.

Patient identifies effective and ineffective coping patterns.

Patient identifies personal strengths that may promote effective coping.

Patient participates in decision-making process.

Other outcomes specific to patient (specify).

Documentation

Specify frequency.

Target date

Specify estimated date of completion.

Nursing interventions
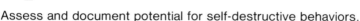

Assess and document potential for self-destructive behaviors.

Encourage patient to verbalize feelings.

Encourage patient to demonstrate feelings without judging.

Encourage patient to request significant persons to visit whenever possible.

Encourage patient to initiate conversations with others.

Assist patient to identify personal strengths.

Encourage patient to express concerns and help solve problems.

Encourage patient involvement in planning care activities.

Encourage patient to participate in activity.

Promote a trusting relationship with patient and family.

Explore available resources with patient and family.

Involve hospital resources in provision of human support for patient and family.

Initiate a patient care conference to review patient's coping mechanisms and to establish a plan of care.

Other interventions specific to patient (specify).

Coping, Ineffective individual

Related to: Dependent behavior, Others specific to patient. (See also preceding diagnosis.)

A condition in which an individual could be unable, or is unable, to maintain his or her usual level of functioning in physical, emotional, or psychological support of self because of actual or perceived changes in the environment

Defining characteristics

Subjective

Expressing lack of confidence in ability to be independent
Making unrealistic requests for assistance with self-care activities
Expressing unwillingness to assume self-care
Expressing anxiety
Expressing apathy
Expressing fear

Objective

Apathy
Regressive behavior
Withdrawal

Outcomes

Patient acknowledges need for independent behavior.
Patient acknowledges awareness of dependent behavior.
Patient follows agreed-upon goals.
Patient demonstrates increased independence.
Patient demonstrates optimal independence.
Patient reports decreased anxiety and fear in independent activities.
Patient demonstrates decreased anxiety and fear in independent activities.
Other outcomes specific to patient (specify).

Documentation
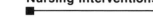

Specify frequency.

Target date

Specify estimated date of completion.

Nursing interventions

Assess and document dependent behaviors, values, and beliefs that interfere with effective coping.

Assist patient to identify dependent/independent behaviors.

Define clear, realistic expectations with patient, promoting independent behaviors.

Encourage patient to verbalize acceptance of changes in behaviors leading to increased independence.

Encourage patient to verbalize increased anxiety and fear regarding independent behaviors.

Encourage and give support to patient's demonstration of independent behaviors.

Provide continuity of patient care through patient assignment and use of care plan.

Initiate a patient care conference to establish goals for patient care, including patient/family members as appropriate.

Maintain consistent assertive approach in care by following agreed-upon care regimen. Set limits and establish contracts with patient. Document those limits and contracts in nurse's notes.

Provide care in an unhurried, supportive, nonjudgmental manner to assist patient to decrease anxiety.

Include the family in the care regimen to encourage their participation in meeting established goals.

Encourage patient to meet/discuss with patients in similar situation in order to learn new ways to cope with situation and to decrease isolation and fear.

Consult with social services to help patient/family progress toward independent behaviors.

Other interventions specific to patient (specify).

Diversional activity deficit

Related to: Boredom, Others specific to patient.

A condition in which an individual experiences, or could experience, insufficient environmental stimulation

Defining characteristics

Subjective

Showing increased dependence on staff
Verbalizing boredom
Complaining of anger
Complaining of not being able to continue with usual activity

Objective

Anger
Flat affect
Increase in daytime sleep
Lability
Restlessness
Disruptive behavior

Outcomes

Patient verbalizes boredom.

Patient identifies activities that may provide stimulation.

Patient verbalizes feelings regarding restrictions imposed by hospitalization.

Patient demonstrates increasing tolerance to circumstances that contribute to boredom.

Patient helps identify activity alternatives.

Other outcomes specific to patient (specify).

Documentation
■——————————————————————————————

Specify frequency.

Target date
■——————————————————————————————

Specify estimated date of completion.

Nursing interventions
■——————————————————————————————

Encourage patient to verbalize feelings and concerns regarding boredom.

Provide appropriate stimuli, e.g., music, games, visitors, and relaxation therapy, to vary monotonous routines and stimulate thought.

Alternate patient care routine, involving patient in plan.

Identify resources, e.g., volunteers and occupational therapists, that would assist patient in recreational activities.

Provide compatible roommate, if possible.

Introduce patient to other patients who have dealt successfully with similar situations.

Encourage family, friends, and significant persons to visit.

Encourage patient to participate in activities of interest that can be provided while hospitalized.

Other interventions specific to patient (specify).

■——————————————————————————————

Family process, Alteration in

Related to: Care of elderly family member, Change in family roles, Complex therapies, Hospitalization, Illness of family member, Others specific to patient/family.

A condition in which a family unit is unable, or could be unable, to maintain its usual level of physical, emotional, or psychological support of each other because of actual or perceived changes in the environment

Defining characteristics

Subjective

Expressing concern regarding disruption of family unit
Expressing concern regarding change in family role expectations
Complaining of altered eating habits
Expressing sleep pattern disruption
Expressing differing expectations
Expressing anger
Expressing anxiety
Expressing inability to accept situation
Expressing depression
Somatic complaints by family members
Stating "I can't cope."

Objective

Absence of family interaction
Entry of elderly family member into home
Identified physical, emotional neglect of patient by family
Interference with nursing/medical care by family
Manipulative behavior
Pacing movements
Verbal hostility among family members
Verbal hostility between family and patient
Verbal hostility between family and staff

Outcomes

Family member/significant other verbalizes anger.

Family member/significant other verbalizes anxiety.

Family member/significant other acknowledges inability to accept situation.

Family member/significant other verbalizes depression.

Family member/significant other verbalizes understanding of the change in family roles.

Family member/significant other identifies coping patterns.

Family member/significant other verbalizes personal strengths.

Family member/significant other identifies decision-making processes.

Family member/significant other participates in decision-making processes regarding posthospital care.

Other outcomes specific to family (specify).

Documentation

Specify frequency.

Target date

Specify estimated date of completion.

Nursing interventions

Assess interaction between patient and family member/significant other, being alert for potentially destructive behaviors.

Encourage family member/significant other to verbalize feelings.

Encourage family member/significant other to demonstrate feelings.

Promote an open, trusting relationship with family member/significant other.

Encourage family member/significant other to visit patient whenever possible. Provide privacy to facilitate family interactions.

Help family member/significant other to identify personal strengths.

Help family member/significant other to identify behaviors that may be interfering with prescribed treatment.

Encourage family member/significant other to participate in patient's activities.

Explore available resources with family member/significant other.

Encourage staff to accept and support the realities of the coping mechanisms of the family member/significant other.

Provide continuity of care by maintaining effective communication between staff members through nurse report, patient care conferences, and care planning.

Initiate a multidisciplinary patient care conference, involving the family and significant others in problem solving and facilitation of communication.

Encourage family member/significant other to express concerns and to help plan posthospital care.

Request social service consultation to help the family determine posthospitalization needs and identify sources of community support.

Facilitate the family's interaction with a financial counselor.

Other interventions specific to family (specify).

Fear

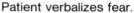

Related to: Disease process, Hospitalization, Invasive medical procedures, Powerlessness, Real or imagined threat to well-being, Surgical procedure, Others specific to patient.

A condition in which an individual could experience, or is experiencing, apprehension caused by a self-identified source. Removal of the source eliminates the apprehension

Defining characteristics

Subjective

Expressing fear
Expressing increased tension
Expressing feelings of panic
Verbalizing feelings of helplessness
Expressing decrease in self-assurance
Identifying source of threat
Identifying source of potential injury
Complaining of dry mouth
Verbalizing need to withdraw from situation

Objective

Nervous behavior
Increased pulse rate
Sweaty palms
Dilated pupils
Increased concentration on identified threat
Decrease in gastrointestinal activity

Outcomes

Patient verbalizes fear.
Patient verbalizes a reduction in fear.
Patient identifies the source of the fear.
Patient identifies behaviors that may reduce fear.
Patient demonstrates behaviors that reduce fear.
Patient identifies behaviors that may eliminate fear.
Patient demonstrates behaviors that eliminate fear.
Other outcomes specific to patient (specify).

Documentation
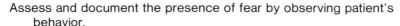

Specify frequency.

Target date

Specify estimated date of completion.

Nursing interventions

Assess and document the presence of fear by observing patient's behavior.

Encourage patient to differentiate between real and imagined threat to well-being by discussing the sources of fear in a supportive, calm manner.

Convey an acceptance of the patient's perception of fear to encourage open communication regarding the source of the fear.

Encourage and assist patient to express the contributing factors that have produced the feelings of fear.

Provide continual verbal and nonverbal reassurances to assist in reducing the patient's fear state.

Remove the source of the patient's fear, if possible.

Provide patient with information regarding procedures and hospital routine as a means of reducing fear.

Provide frequent, positive reinforcement in response to patient's demonstration of behaviors that may reduce or eliminate fear.

Confer with physician regarding patient's fear in order to encourage a discussion between the patient and physician.

Ensure continuity in plan of care through initiation of a multidisciplinary patient care conference, and regularity in patient assignment.

Assess need for social service and/or crisis intervention services. Provide this service to assist in the reduction of the patient's apprehension, if necessary.

Other interventions specific to patient (specify).

Fluid volume, Alteration in: *Excess*

Related to: Specific to patient.

A condition in which an individual experiences, or could experience, an excessive accumulation of body fluids

Defining characteristics

Subjective

Complaining of swelling
Complaining of shortness of breath
Complaining of difficulty in movement, ambulation
Complaining of feeling agitated or restless

Objective

Weight gain
Increased or decreased blood pressure
Increased pulse rate
Increased respiratory rate
Decreased urine output
Intake greater than output
Shortness of breath
Adventitious lung sounds
Neck vein distention
Increased abdominal distention (ascites)
Swelling of dependent body part
Taut, shiny skin
Pitting edema
Change in level of consciousness
Abnormal laboratory values

Outcomes

Patient's edema decreases toward normal limits for patient.

Patient's target weight is achieved. Specify target weight.

Patient's skin integrity is maintained.

Patient verbalizes understanding of fluid and dietary restrictions.

Patient's vital signs are within normal limits for patient. Specify normal limits.

Other outcomes specific to patient (specify).

Documentation

Specify frequency.

Target date

Specify estimated date of completion.

Nursing interventions

Assess and document presence or absence of peripheral pulse, temperature, capillary refill, color,and edema in extremities q ____.

Assess and document vital signs q ____.

Assess and document adventitious lung sounds q ____.

Assess and document pulmonary and cardiovascular problems as indicated by increased respiratory distress, increased pulse rate, increased blood pressure, and decreased urine output. Notify physician of assessment.

Assess, palpate, and document presence of edema on scale from 1+ − 4+. Specify location.

Assess and document presence of sacral edema q ____.

Assess and document abdominal girth q ____.

Weigh q ____.

Record input and output q ____.

Assess for balanced input and output.

Assess and document effects of medications, e.g., steroids, diuretics, on edema.

Elevate extremities to increase venous return.

Change position q ____.

Maintain patient's fluid restriction.

Instruct and encourage dietary restrictions within limitations of diet.

Other interventions specific to patient (specify).

Fluid volume deficit

Related to: Abnormal fluid loss (specify), Others specific to patient. (See also following diagnosis.)

A condition in which an individual experiences, or could experience, an excessive loss of body fluids

Defining characteristics

Subjective	Objective
Complaining of fatigue	Increased pulse rate
Complaining of thirst	Hypotension
Expressing confusion	Elevated body temperature
	Urine output less than 30cc/hour
	Increased specific gravity of urine
	Dry mucous membranes
	Poor skin turgor
	Output greater than intake
	Weight loss
	Increased loss of body fluids from gastro-intestinal tract
	Increased loss of body fluids from surgical incision or other wounds
	Hemorrhage
	Increased urine output from disease or medical therapy
	Abnormal laboratory values, such as Na+, K+, hemoglobin, hematocrit, FBS, and BUN
	Confusion

Outcomes

Patient is oriented to person, place, and time.

Patient is free of nausea and vomiting.

Patient has normal skin turgor.

Patient has moist mucous membranes.

Patient's urine output is not less than 30cc/hour.

Patient's vital signs are within normal limits for patient. Specify normal limits.

Patient's intake and output are balanced.

Patient maintains his or her weight. Specify admission weight.

Patient's serum electrolytes are within normal range for patient. Specify normal range.

Outcomes *(continued)*

Patient's hemoglobin and packed cell volume are within normal range for patient. Specify normal range.

Patient's intake is maintained at _____ cc fluids/24 hours.

Patient's skin remains warm and dry.

Patient is free of sudden restlessness.

Other outcomes specific to patient (specify).

Documentation

Specify frequency.

Target date

Specify estimated date of completion.

Nursing interventions

Assess and document skin turgor and mucous membranes q _____ as parameters for adequate hydration.

Assess and document specific gravity and color of urine q _____.

Assess and document color, amount, and frequency of emesis, diarrhea, and other drainage.

Assess and document vital signs q _____.

Assess and document orientation to person, place, and time q _____.

Assess and document dressing changes to evaluate fluid loss through wounds.

Assess and document skin temperature, dryness, and color.

Assess and document intake and output.

Assess and document back of throat for active bleeding, using tongue blade and flashlight.

Weigh patient q _____.

Encourage oral fluid intake. Specify amount to be drunk in 24 hours, quantifying desired intake during the day, evening, and night shifts.

Review electrolytes and report any abnormalities, especially Na+, K+, Chloride, BUN, and creatinine.

Confer with physician regarding need for parenteral electrolyte replacement therapy.

Report and document output over _____ cc.

Report and document output under _____ cc.

Include patient in planning of care activities.

Other interventions specific to patient (specify).

Fluid volume deficit

Related to: Decreased fluid intake, Others specific to patient. (See also preceding diagnosis.)

A condition in which an individual experiences, or could experience, homeostatic changes as a consequence of inadequate fluid intake

Defining characteristics

Subjective

Complaining of thirst
Complaining of fatigue
Expressing confusion

Objective

Hypotension
Elevated body temperature
Urine output less than 30cc/hour
Increased specific gravity of urine
Dry mucous membranes
Poor skin turgor
Output greater than intake
Weight loss
Abnormal laboratory values

Outcomes

Patient has normal skin turgor.

Patient has moist mucous membranes.

Patient's urine output is not less than 30cc/hour.

Patient maintains his or her weight. Specify admission weight.

Patient reports no thirst.

Patient reports no weakness.

Serum electrolytes are within normal range for patient. Specify normal range.

Patient's intake is maintained at ____ cc fluids/24 hours.

Other outcomes specific to patient (specify).

Documentation
—

Specify frequency.

Target date
—

Specify estimated date of completion.

Nursing interventions
—

Assess and document skin turgor and mucous membranes q ____ as parameters for adequate hydration.

Assess for contributing factors that may aggravate dehydration, such as medications, fever, stress, medical orders.

Measure and document input and output q ____ .

Assess and document specific gravity and color of urine q ____ .

Weigh patient q ____ .

Instruct patient to inform nurse of thirst.

Offer fluid of patient's choice at bedside.

Encourage fluid intake. Specify amount to be drunk in 24 hours, quantifying desired intake during the day shift, evening shift, and night shift.

Report and document output over ____ cc.

Report and document output under ____ cc.

Evaluate presence of weakness during activity and pace according to patient's tolerance.

Review electrolytes and report any abnormalities, especially Na+, K+, chloride, BUN, and creatinine.

Confer with physician regarding need for parenteral electrolyte replacement therapy.

Other interventions specific to patient (specify).

—

Grieving

Related to: Actual loss, Anticipated loss, Perceived loss, Others specific to patient.

A condition in which an individual experiences, or could experience, a normal emotional response to an actual, anticipated, or perceived loss, for instance, of a significant person, ideals, a body part, status, or an object

Defining characteristics

Subjective

Expressing anger
Verbalizing depression
Expressing inability to accept situation
Expressing grief
Expressing sorrow
Verbalizing need to bargain
Verbalizing acceptance of loss

Objective

Crying
Medical diagnosis of terminal illness
Medical diagnosis of chronic illness
Loss of extremity, body part
Demonstrated change in eating
    behavior
Withdrawal

Outcomes

Patient verbalizes grief.

Patient shares grief with significant person.

Patient verbalizes perceptions of loss as it relates to self.

Patient identifies his or her role in decision-making process.

Patient uses available resources.

Other outcomes specific to patient (specify).

Documentation
■————————————————————

Specify frequency.

Target date
■————————————————————

Specify estimated date of completion.

Nursing interventions
■————————————————————

Assess and document the presence and source of patient's grief.
Establish a trusting relationship with patient and family.
Encourage patient to express grief.
Evaluate verbal and nonverbal communication as they relate to grieving process.
Provide a safe, secure, and private environment to facilitate patient/family grieving process.
Recognize and reinforce the strength of each family member.
Explain to patient/family the necessary care activities, allowing for flexibility in schedule of activities.
Demonstrate respect for patient's culture, religion, race, and values as patient expresses grief.
Discuss with patient/family the impact of the loss on the family unit and its functioning.
Find support among peers, recognizing the health care provider's own limitations, and using others to provide needed patient care activities.
Provide literature on hospital- and community-based programs to patient and family.
Explore available community resources, such as self-help groups, with patient/family.
Initiate a patient care conference to review patient/family needs related to their stage of the grieving process, and to establish a plan of care.
Other interventions specific to patient (specify).

■————————————————————

Health maintenance, Alterations in

Related to: Health beliefs, Others specific to patient.

A condition in which an individual is unable or unwilling, or could be unable or unwilling, to identify, to learn, or to maintain optimal wellness

Defining characteristics

Subjective

Reporting limited use of health care agencies and personnel

Expressing desire to improve health behaviors

Reporting limited use of preventative health measures

Having history of nontreated, chronic symptoms of disease process

Objective

Hypertension

Body lesions

Obesity

Smoking

Unclean physical appearance

Elevated serum glucose

Outcomes

Patient verbalizes knowledge of adverse effects of previous health beliefs.

Patient acknowledges necessity for assistance after discharge.

Patient verbalizes willingness to follow nursing/medical regimen.

Patient demonstrates knowledge of preventative health measures.

Other outcomes specific to patient (specify).

Documentation
■─────────────────────────────────

Specify frequency.

Target date
■─────────────────────────────────

Specify estimated date of completion.

Nursing interventions
■─────────────────────────────────

Initiate a discussion of health beliefs with patient/family.

Provide a nonjudgmental environment in which patient/family can share health beliefs.

Encourage discussion of preventative health measures specific to patient needs, such as dietary changes, cessation of smoking, stress reduction, implementation of exercise program, etc.

Evaluate patient/family ability to perform learned skills after discharge by requesting a return demonstration.

Offer information on community resources specific to health maintenance needs of patient/family.

Initiate a multidisciplinary patient care conference to discuss health maintenance needs with patient and family.

Other interventions specific to patient (specify).

■─────────────────────────────────

Home maintenance management,
Impaired

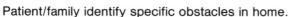

Related to: Disease of family member other than patient, Home environment obstacles, Inadequate support system, Insufficient family organization or planning, Others specific to patient.

A condition in which an individual or family is unable, or could be unable, to maintain a safe home environment due to physical, financial, emotional, or psychological obstacles

Defining characteristics

Subjective

Patient espressing inability to
 "manage at home"
Family expressing environmental
 obstacles inhibiting home care
Family expressing financial obstacles
 inhibiting home care
Family expressing inability to cope
 with patient at home
Family expressing inability to maintain
 hygienic home environment
Family expressing need for external
 support system to facilitate care
 of patient at home
Family requesting assistance in care
 of patient at home

Outcomes

Patient/family identify specific obstacles in home.

Patient/family verbalize knowledge of available resources.

Patient/family verbalize financial constraints.

Patient/family establish specific plan for home health maintenance.

Patient/family demonstrate understanding of disease process and its
 effect on the home situation.

Patient/family demonstrate management of home self-care activities.

Patient/family verbalize awareness of constraints on home situation
 because of illness of family member other than patient.

Patient/family verbalize present family organizational and functional
 strengths and weaknesses.

Other outcomes specific to patient (specify).

Documentation

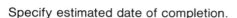

Specify frequency.

Target date

Specify estimated date of completion.

Nursing interventions

Assess and document need for discharge planning/social worker, using information from patient and family.

Initiate discussion with patient/family about health status of all family members, as illness of other family members may affect home maintenance management.

Help patient/family identify obstacles in home that may impede home health maintenance.

Help patient/family identify strengths in family unit as well as support systems that will assist home health maintenance.

Instruct and support patient/family in assuming health maintenance activities while in hospital.

Contact discharge planning/social worker to facilitate home maintenance management.

Establish realistic plan for home management with discharge planning/social worker.

Involve family/significant person in all planning activities.

Provide patient/family with written material regarding home health maintenance.

Listen, without judgment, to the realities of the home situation.

Assess for accurate feedback by requesting a return demonstration to ensure adequate teaching for home health maintenance.

Assess and document patient's/family's progress toward learning.

Assess and document need for postdischarge follow-through, with clinic visits or support groups.

Other interventions specific to patient (specify).

Injury, Potential for

Related to: Hypotension, Motor deficit, Psychomotor hyperactivity, Sensory deficit, Substance intoxication, Others specific to patient.

A condition in which an individual experiences, or could experience, an injury because of mental or physical limitations, and/or hazards in the environment

Defining characteristics

Subjective

Verbalizing lack of knowledge about safety
Reporting a hearing deficit
Reporting a visual impairment
Complaining of vertigo
Reporting a history of falls/injuries
Reporting numbness or lack of sensation

Objective

Broken skin
Broken bone or other injury
History of seizures
Disorientation
Confusion
Tremors
Agitation
Environmental changes
Incorrect use of mobility aids
Unsteady gait
Debilitation

Outcomes

Patient avoids physical injury.
Patient achieves his or her own optimal activity level without injury.
Patient demonstrates understanding of limitations on activity.
Patient verbalizes need for assistance.
Patient reports any dizziness or unsteadiness during activities.
Other outcomes specific to patient (specify).

Documentation

Specify frequency.

Target date

Specify estimated date of completion.

Nursing interventions
∎————————————————————————————

Assess and document patient's motor deficit.

Assess and document patient's sensory deficit.

Assess and document for etiology of motor/sensory deficit, such as medications, hypoxia, or electrolyte imbalance.

Assess and document degree of intoxication to determine safety needs of patient.

Assess and document degree of disorientation to determine safety needs of patient.

Confer with physician regarding medications that may improve or correct motor/sensory deficit. Assess and document effectiveness of medication following administration.

Use safety measures, such as foam mattress, foot cradle, heel and elbow pads, to prevent injury.

Keep frequently used items within patient's reach.

Encourage patient's use of hearing aids, glasses, etc.

Reorient patient to reality and immediate environment when necessary.

Encourage patient to request assistance with ambulation.

Keep environment clear of obstructions.

Check patient for presence of constrictive clothing, cuts, burns, bruises.

Place patient in a room near the nurses' station.

Provide an electric razor for shaving.

Use soft restraints that allow optimal movement to prevent injury, if needed.

Do not support patient's hallucinations or otherwise contribute to disorientation.

Remove potentially harmful objects, including smoking materials, from patient's room.

Ensure that patient is not alone while smoking.

Discuss with patient/family necessity for use of soft restraints, assistance with ambulation, and use of preventative equipment to ensure patient safety.

Other interventions specific to patient (specify).

∎————————————————————————————

Knowledge deficit

Related to: Limited understanding of disease process, Limited understanding of prescribed treatment, Others specific to patient.

A condition in which the individual/family experiences, or could experience, an inability to learn, comprehend, or demonstrate knowledge of health care measures necessary to maintain or improve wellness

Defining characteristics

Subjective

Patient/family expressing limited understanding of disease process

Patient/family expressing limited knowledge of prescribed treatment

Patient/family expressing desire to learn skill or aspects of prescribed treatment

Patient/family expressing lack of comprehension of prescribed treatment due to emotional/psychological barriers to acceptance of health situation

Patient/family refusing to learn skill or prescribed treatment

Objective

Demonstrated cognitive deficit of patient/family

Demonstrated limited skill in performance of necessary skill or treatment

Lack of comprehension of prescribed treatment or skill due to emotional/psychological barriers to acceptance of health situation

Demonstrated sensory deficit of patient/family that may inhibit learning

Outcomes

Patient verbalizes perception of health status.

Patient identifies need for additional information regarding prescribed treatment.

Patient verbalizes understanding of need for support person to ensure optimal treatment regimen.

Patient demonstrates ability to follow prescribed regimen.

Other outcomes specific to patient/family (specify).

Documentation

Specify frequency.

Target date

Specify estimated date of completion.

Nursing interventions

Assess and document patient's level of understanding of prescribed treatment.

Assess and document patient's readiness to learn treatment regimen.

Plan with patient and physician adjustment in treatment to facilitate patient's ability to follow prescribed treatment.

Provide teaching at patient's level of understanding, repeating information as necessary. Be realistic.

Interact with patient in nonjudgmental manner to facilitate learning.

Involve support person/significant person in teaching process.

Check for accurate feedback to ensure patient understands prescribed treatment.

Document patient's process in nurse's notes.

Provide literature specific to patient's learning needs.

Reinforce teaching as necessary, using multiple teaching approaches, return demonstrations, verbal and written feedback.

Provide information on community resources that will help patient maintain treatment regimen.

Other interventions specific to patient (specify).

Mobility, Impaired physical

Related to: Decreased strength and endurance, Musculoskeletal impairment, Neuromuscular impairment, Others specific to patient.

A condition in which the individual experiences, or could experience, limitations of independent physical movement. Specify one of these levels*:

Level I: Requires use of equipment or device.

Level II: Requires assistance, supervision, or teaching from others.

Level III: Requires help from others and equipment or device.

Level IV: Is dependent and does not participate in movement.

Defining characteristics

Subjective

Expressing instability or weakness
Expressing fear of falling during ambulation
Expressing fear of pain during movement

Objective

Impaired motor coordination
Limited movement due to medical condition or treatment regimen, such as traction, bed rest, restraints, casts, edema
Limited range of motion

Outcomes

Patient acknowledges limitations in strength and endurance.

Patient maintains or increases strength and endurance.

Patient demonstrates ability to cope with limitations.

Patient shows knowledge of safety measures that minimize potential for injury.

Patient demonstrates safety measures that minimize potential for injury.

Patient performs active range-of-motion exercises.

Patient operates mobility equipment effectively.

Patient demonstrates safe transfer technique from bed to wheelchair or commode.

Patient performs prescribed exercises independently.

Patient demonstrates ability to use aids to mobility.

Patient walks with use of ambulation aids.

Patient increases ambulation to gain optimal level of independence.

Other outcomes specific to patient (specify).

* Gordon, M.: *Manual of nursing diagnosis 1984–1985.* New York: McGraw-Hill, 1985.

Documentation

Specify frequency.

Target date

Specify estimated date of completion.

Nursing interventions

Assess and document the degree to which patient's mobility is impaired.

Assess and document the number of personnel needed for transfers.

Assess the patient's learning needs regarding safe transfer.

Develop and document a plan for mobility and transfer prior to activity.

Develop and document a plan for maintaining or increasing muscle strength and endurance.

Discuss with patient/family the patient's limitations in mobility, and enlist the family's assistance during activity.

Instruct the patient and family in safe use of aids to mobility.

Instruct and encourage the patient in active range-of-motion exercises to maintain or develop muscle strength and endurance.

Instruct the patient in safe transfer from bed to wheelchair or commode and encourage the patient's attempts.

Instruct patient regarding weight-bearing status.

Instruct patient regarding correct body alignment.

Instruct and encourage patient to use a trapeze and/or weights to strengthen and maintain upper extremity strength.

Encourage patient to verbalize limitations in strength and endurance.

Provide positive verbal reinforcement during patient activities.

Encourage patient/family to view physical limitations realistically.

Use occupational/physical therapists as resources in planning patient care activities.

Assess need for home health agency assistance and need for durable medical equipment.

Document patient's level of performance in activities, noting any increase or decrease in strength and endurance.

Other interventions specific to patient (specify).

Noncompliance

Related to: Dysfunctional relationship with health care providers, Negative consequence of treatment regimen, Negative perception of treatment regimen, Others specific to patient.

A condition in which the individual chooses not to adhere to the recommended treatment plan

Defining characteristics

Subjective

Patient or family reporting patient's noncompliance with treatment regimen

Patient reporting treatment is in conflict with lifestyle

Complaining of exacerbation of signs and symptoms due to nonadherence to medication regimen

Complaining of side-effects of prescribed medications

Taking nontherapeutic dosages of medication

Expressing unwillingness to follow plan of care while hospitalized

Expressing dissatisfaction with health care providers

Expressing dissatisfaction with health care setting

Failing to keep appointments

Outcomes

Patient verbalizes feelings about relationship with health care providers.

Patient identifies anticipated or experienced consequences of treatment regimen that led to noncompliant behavior.

Patient verbalizes feelings about hospitalization.

Patient does not abuse health care providers physically or verbally.

Patient participates in agreed-upon plan of care while hospitalized.

Patient identifies physical/emotional/cultural factors that precipitated noncompliance with treatment regimen.

Other outcomes specific to patient (specify).

Documentation
▆

Specify frequency.

Target date
▆

Specify estimated date of completion.

Nursing interventions
▆

Assess and document patient's understanding of the treatment regimen as a baseline for determining noncompliant behavior.

Establish a therapeutic, nonjudgmental environment in which the patient can express feelings and concerns about hospitalization and his or her relationship to health care providers.

Involve the patient in determining what behavior constitutes compliance.

Give positive reinforcement for compliance to encourage ongoing positive behaviors.

Develop a written contract with the patient, and evaluate compliant behaviors on a continuing basis.

Inform patient that physical/verbal abuse is not acceptable and will not be tolerated.

Discuss with patient/family those physical/emotional/cultural factors that may have precipitated noncompliance with treatment regimen.

Use hospital resources and other staff members to confront patient with his or her nonacceptable behavior.

Initiate patient care conference to establish consistency in approach to patient. Document approach in nursing care plan.

Evaluate patient's need for emotional support from hospital resources/ social worker.

Provide emotional support to family member/significant other to help them maintain a positive relationship with patient.

Provide and reinforce information regarding treatment regimen so that patient/family understand the necessity of following prescribed treatment.

Consult with physician about possible alteration in medical regimen to encourage patient compliance.

Other interventions specific to patient (specify).

▆

Nutrition, Alteration in:
Less than body requirements

■━━━━━━━━━━━━━━━━━━━━━━━━━━━━━━

Related to: Difficulty swallowing, Others specific to patient. (See also two following diagnoses.)

A condition in which the individual fails to ingest, or could fail to ingest, the nutrients necessary to meet metabolic needs

Defining characteristics
■━━━━━━━━━━━━━━━━━━━━━━━━━━━━━━

Subjective

Complaining of difficulty swallowing
Complaining of pain on swallowing
Stating inability to consume all but
    certain foods

Objective

Impaired ability to swallow
Coughing during ingestion of liquid
Refusal to eat
Lack of gag reflex
Ulcerated oral mucosa

Outcomes
■━━━━━━━━━━━━━━━━━━━━━━━━━━━━━━

Patient ingests nutrients orally.
Patient swallows without choking.
Patient swallows without pain.
Patient eats prescribed diet.

Documentation
■───

Specify frequency.

Target date
■───

Specify estimated date of completion.

Nursing interventions
■───

Assess and document etiology of swallowing difficulty.

Carefully observe attempts to swallow.

Reassure patient and provide calm atmosphere during meals.

Have suction catheters available at bedside, and suction during meals, as needed.

Place patient in position that facilitates swallowing.

Place food on unaffected side of mouth to facilitate swallowing of food.

Prepare patient for meals, provide privacy, and assist in an unhurried manner.

Use syringe, if necessary, when feeding patient to facilitate swallowing.

Identify and document foods patient can tolerate.

Document food intake; use calorie counts.

Document feeding technique.

Confer with physician regarding need for nutritional tube feedings/TPN so that adequate calorie intake is maintained.

Have occupational therapist/dietitian counsel patient on meal planning and swallowing techniques.

Other interventions specific to patient (specify).

■───

Nutrition, Alteration in:
Less than body requirements

Related to: High metabolic states, Inadequate nutrition, Loss of appetite, Others specific to patient. (Also see following and preceding diagnoses.)

A condition in which an individual fails to ingest or absorb, or could fail to ingest or absorb, the nutrients necessary to meet metabolic needs

Defining characteristics

Subjective

Complaining of loss of appetite
Complaining of loss of appetite due to medications
Complaining of loss of interest in food
Complaining of inability to eat
Complaining of indigestion/stomach cramps, nausea, vomiting
Verbalizing depression
Family expressing concern about limited intake of food by patient

Objective

Body weight 20% or more under ideal for height and frame
Refusal to eat
Weight loss
Abnormal laboratory values, such as transferrin, albumin, electrolytes

Outcomes

Patient maintains weight at ____ kg.

Patient verbalizes willingness to follow diet.

Patient is free of nausea and/or vomiting.

Patient shows increased appetite.

Patient eats and drinks predetermined amount.

Other outcomes specific to patient (specify).

Documentation
■─────────────────────────────────────

Specify frequency.

Target date
■─────────────────────────────────────

Specify estimated date of completion.

Nursing interventions
■─────────────────────────────────────

Assess and document bowel sounds and abdominal distention q ____.

Assess and document laboratory values, especially transferrin, albumin, and electrolytes.

Assess and document medications that may be contributing to loss of appetite.

Weigh patient q ____.

Assist patient with meals, as needed.

Ensure pleasant surroundings during meals.

Involve patient in a diet plan, including time of meals and eating environment.

Confer with dietitian to establish caloric requirements, using anthropometric measurements, especially for patients with high energy needs, such as those with burns, trauma, fever, and wounds, as well as postoperative patients.

Have dietitian talk with patient about likes, dislikes, and schedule of meals.

Ensure that food is served at appropriate temperature.

Give positive feedback to patient who shows increased appetite.

Document amount and calorie count of food ingested.

Instruct patient to notify nurse of nausea.

Medicate nauseated patients consistently, on a set schedule, to prevent nausea.

Document color and amount of vomit and frequency of emesis.

Identify factors, such as depression, that may contribute to loss of appetite.

Encourage family member/significant person to bring food of patient's preference from home.

Confer with physician regarding need for nutritional tube feedings/TPN so that adequate calorie intake is maintained.

Other interventions specific to patient (specify).

■─────────────────────────────────────

Nutrition, Alteration in:
Less than body requirements
▬══════════════════════════

Related to: Nausea and/or vomiting, Others specific to patient. (See also two preceding diagnoses.)

A condition in which an individual ingests, or could ingest, a diet that does not meet metabolic requirements because of a decreased desire for, and/or an inability to tolerate, food

Defining characteristics
■─────────────────────────

Subjective

Complaining of nausea
Complaining that certain odors
    increase nausea
Requesting antiemetics

Objective

Emesis
Limited oral intake
Refusing to eat

Outcomes
■─────────────────────────

Patient states that nausea is decreasing.
Patient vomits with less frequency.
Patient is free of aspiration.
Patient eats and retains prescribed diet.

Documentation

Specify frequency.

Target date

Specify estimated date of completion.

Nursing interventions

Assess and document presence of bowel sounds and abdominal distention.

Assess and document need for parenteral/enteral nutrition.

Assess and document factors that may precipitate nausea and vomiting.

Instruct patient to inform nurse of nausea.

Document presence or absence of nausea and/or vomiting.

Document color and amount of vomit and frequency of vomiting.

Position patient during meals, and for 30 minutes following meals, to prevent aspiration.

Keep suction equipment available.

Instruct patient in slow, deep breathing and voluntary swallowing to decrease nausea and/or vomiting.

Offer cool, wet washcloth to be placed on forehead or back of neck.

Reassure and support patient during episodes of emesis.

Minimize unpleasant sights and odors near patient.

Offer oral hygiene q ____.

Administer antiemetics, as needed. Assess and document effectiveness.

Other interventions specific to patient (specify).

Nutrition, Alteration in:
More than body requirements

Related to: Ingestion of intake greater than metabolic requirements, Others specific to patient.

A condition in which an individual weighs, or could weigh, 10%–20% more than his or her ideal weight, possibly with negative effects on health

Defining characteristics

Subjective

Expressing an altered body image
Expressing need for emotional
    rewards through food
Espressing depression, stress
Expressing boredom
Verbalizing unhealthy learned eating
    habits and behaviors

Objective

Body weight 10%–20% above ideal
    for height and frame
Sedentary lifestyle
Decreasing metabolic requirements
Medications that stimulate appetite
Requesting large portions at meals
Endocrine disorders

Outcomes

Patient acknowledges weight problem.

Patient verbalizes desire to lose weight.

Patient identifies eating habits and behaviors that produce weight gain.

Patient identifies eating habits and behaviors that produce weight loss.

Patient identifies activities that increase metabolic requirements.

Patient identifies physical/emotional benefits of weight loss.

Patient acknowledges need to participate in a structured weight loss program.

Patient participates in nutritional counseling.

Other outcomes specific to patient (specify).

Documentation

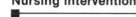

Specify frequency.

Target date

Specify estimated date of completion.

Nursing interventions

Assess on admission for medical conditions that may contribute to weight gain.

Request information from patient/family regarding patient's current eating habits and behaviors that may contribute to weight gain or to the maintenance of current weight status.

Request information from patient/family regarding patient's current activity level that correlates to the patient's metabolic needs.

Request dietitian to perform nutritional assessment, including triceps skin fold measurement, height and weight measurement, and diet history.

Confer with dietitian to establish weight loss program that includes dietary management and takes activity limitations into account.

Help patient identify somatic complaints that may be due to present weight status.

Confer with physician regarding weight loss contract that may begin while patient is hospitalized.

Provide frequent positive reinforcement for such behavior changes as weight loss, maintenance of dietary regimen, improved eating behaviors.

Identify family member or friend who might support and encourage weight loss efforts after discharge.

Provide information about available community resources, such as weight loss groups, dietary counseling, health clubs.

Other interventions specific to patient (specify).

Oral mucous membranes, Alteration in

■══

Related to: Insufficient oral hygiene, Stomatitis, Others specific to patient.

A condition in which an individual experiences, or could experience, an inflammation and/or irritation of the mucosa of the mouth

Defining characteristics
■──

Subjective

Complaining of mouth pain
Complaining of discomfort caused by
  ingesting hot or cold foods

Objective

Irritation or inflammation of oral
  mucosa
Dry mouth
Bleeding gums
Bad breath
Coated tongue
Dry, cracked lips

Outcomes
■──

Patient maintains intact oral mucosa.

Patient is free of irritation and inflammation of oral mucosa.

Patient has no oral discomfort when ingesting foods and fluids.

Patient maintains optimal nutrition and hydration.

Patient has no increase in mucosal irritation and inflammation.

Patient performs essential oral hygiene according to prescribed instruction.

Other outcomes specific to patient (specify).

Documentation
▪———————————————————————————————

Specify frequency.

Target date
▪———————————————————————————————

Specify estimated date of completion.

Nursing interventions
▪———————————————————————————————

Assess and document patient's oral mucosa for irritation and inflammation.

Assess and document patient's understanding of need for oral care and ability to perform oral care.

Assess and document patient's tolerance to extremes in food temperatures and seasonings that might increase discomfort.

Assist patient during meals, as needed.

Identify substances that irritate oral mucosa, such as tobacco, alcohol, food, medications.

Use toothettes or soft child's toothbrush, bulb syringe, or suction catheter, which do not irritate oral mucosa.

Provide mouth care prior to meals and q ____ hours to ensure optimal oral hygiene and adequate nutrition.

Plan meals with dietitian to ensure optimal nutrition and hydration.

Confer with physician regarding an order for antifungal mouth wash or oral topical anesthetic as adjuncts to oral hygiene, if fungal infection exists.

Clean dentures after each meal.

Instruct patient/family in oral care routine.

Other interventions specific to patient (specify).

▪———————————————————————————————

Powerlessness

Related to: Disease process, Hospitalization, Others specific to patient.

A condition in which an individual experiences, or could experience, a feeling of insufficient control, influence, and/or authority over the immediate environment

Defining characteristics

Subjective

Complaining of increased dependence
Expressing anger
Verbalizing inability to accept situation
Verbalizing lack of control over environment
Verbalizing lack of control over self-care
Verbalizing lack of control over disease

Outcomes

Patient identifies factors that contribute to a sense of powerlessness.
Patient verbalizes feeling control over environment.
Patient verbalizes feeling control over his or her plan of care.
Patient participates in decision making regarding plan of care.
Other outcomes specific to patient (specify).

Documentation

Specify frequency.

Target date

Specify estimated date of completion.

Nursing interventions

Assess nonverbal indicators of powerlessness such as anger, apathy, listlessness, and depression.

Encourage patient to express feelings of powerlessness.

Help patient to identify factors that may contribute to powerlessness.

Establish a trusting relationship with patient through continuity of care.

Include patient in decision making about care routine.

Provide care in a nonjudgmental, nonauthoritative manner.

Discuss with patient realistic options in care, providing explanations for options.

Document the plan of care as agreed upon by the nurse and patient in the nursing care plan.

Document assessment and effects of therapeutic care in nurse's notes.

Explain the rationale for any deviation in the plan of care to patient.

Provide flexibility in care regimen as indicated by patient's expression of need to alter plan of care.

Initiate a multidisciplinary patient care conference to discuss the patient care routine and factors that contribute to the patient's powerlessness.

Other interventions specific to patient (specify).

Respiratory functions, Alteration in:
Airway clearance, ineffective

■

Related to: Specific to patient.

A condition in which an individual experiences, or could experience, the loss of a patent airway

Defining characteristics
■

Subjective

Complaining of shortness of breath
Expressing anxiety

Objective

Restlessness
Shortness of breath
Abnormal breath sounds, such as
    rales, rhonchi, wheezes
Abnormal blood gases
Change in respiratory rate
Inability to expectorate
Cough
Cyanosis
Decreased or absent breath sounds
    in posterior chest

Outcomes
■

Patient is free of respiratory distress.
Patient is able to expectorate secretions effectively.
Patient achieves optimal pulmonary function.
Other outcomes specific to patient (specify).

Documentation
■

Specify frequency.

Target date
■

Specify estimated date of completion.

Nursing interventions
■

Auscultate and document assessment of lung fields q ____.

Assess and document need for percussion and/or supportive equipment.

Assess and document administration of oxygen and its effectiveness, if ordered.

Observe and document color, consistency, and amount of sputum.

Assess and document trends in arterial blood gases, and notify physician of abnormalities.

Correlate all assessment data, document, and report any changes.

Initiate vigorous pulmonary toilet, which may include percussion, postural drainage, coughing, and deep breathing.

Instruct patient in coughing techniques that facilitate the expectoration of secretions.

Maintain adequate hydration to decrease viscosity of secretions.

Encourage physical activity to promote movement of secretions.

Assess patient's lung sounds, respiratory rate, and production of sputum as indicators of effective use of supportive equipment.

Explain proper use of supportive equipment (O_2, suction, spirometer, IPPB).

Inform patient and family that smoking is prohibited in room.

Utilize suction catheter in the nasopharyngeal/oropharyngeal space to facilitate expectoration of secretions.

Apply suction q ____. Be sure to hyperoxygenate with resuscitator bag prior to suctioning endotracheal tube or tracheostomy.

Other interventions specific to patient (specify).

■

Respiratory functions, Alteration in:
Breathing pattern, ineffective

■

Related to: Specific to patient.

A condition in which an individual experiences, or could experience, inadequate inspiratory and/or expiratory movement of air through the alveoli

Defining characteristics
■

Subjective	Objective
Complaining of anxiety	Dyspnea
Complaining of fatigue	Hyperventilation or hypoventilation
Complaining of inability to breathe effectively	Mouth breathing
	Nasal flaring
Expressing need for supplemental oxygen	Shortness of breath
	Periods of apnea
Complaining of inability to get enough sleep	Tachycardia
	Increased or decreased blood pressure
	Orthopnea, paroxysmal nocturnal dyspnea
	Use of accessory muscles for breathing
	Abnormal blood gases

Outcomes
■

Patient is free of respiratory distress.

Patient demonstrates normal respiratory pattern.

Patient requests breathing assistance when needed.

Patient demonstrates effective breathing pattern.

Arterial blood gases are within normal limits for patient.

Patient achieves optimal pulmonary function.

Patient demonstrates optimal gas exchange with assistance of mechanical ventilator.

Other outcomes specific to patient (specify).

Documentation
■

Specify frequency.

Target date
■

Specify estimated date of completion.

Nursing interventions

Assess and document presence or absence of breath sounds, anterior and posterior, noting rales, rhonchi, wheezes, diminished breath sounds, and absence of breath sounds, splinting and/or abnormal chest wall movement.

Assess and document respiratory pattern, including rate, depth, rhythm q ____.

Assess and document for cyanosis and use of accessory muscles. Position for optimal breathing q ____.

Assess and document effect of medication on respiratory status.

Assess and document degree and characteristics of pain that may inhibit respiratory excursion.

Assess and document location and extent of crepitus over rib cage.

Assess and document lung sounds, respiratory rate, and production of sputum as indicators of effective use of supportive equipment.

Review arterial blood gas results and correlate with clinical condition.

Correlate all assessment data, document, and report any changes.

Instruct patient to notify nurse at onset of ineffective breathing pattern.

Reassure patient during periods of respiratory distress.

Encourage slow abdominal breathing during periods of respiratory distress.

Stay with patient during episodes of acute respiratory distress.

Turn, cough, and deep breathe q ____.

Instruct patient in coughing techniques to expel secretions.

Avoid medications that depress respiratory function.

Administer pain medications to restore optimal respiratory pattern, as needed.

Initiate vigorous pulmonary toilet, which may include percussion, postural drainage, coughing, and deep breathing

Explain proper use of supportive equipment (O_2, suction, spirometer, IPPB).

Maintain low flow of oxygen by nasal cannula or mask.

Inform patient and family that smoking is prohibited in room.

Instruct patient in relaxation techniques to improve breathing pattern.

Apply suction to the nasopharyngeal/oropharyngeal space to facilitate the expectoration of secretions.

Apply suction q ____. Be sure to hyperoxygenate with resuscitator bag prior to suctioning endotracheal tube or tracheostomy.

Keep trach tube at bedside.

Synchronize patient's breathing pattern with ventilator rate.

Observe and document bilateral chest expansion of patient on ventilator.

Other interventions specific to patient (specify).

Respiratory functions, Alteration in:
Gas exchange, impaired

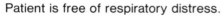

Related to: Disease process, Others specific to patient.

A condition in which an individual experiences, or could experience, an impairment of CO_2 transport from the alveoli to the vascular system

Defining characteristics

Subjective

Complaining of fatigue
Complaining of shortness of breath
Expressing need for supplemental
   oxygen

Objective

Restlessness
Tachycardia
Sensory changes
Confusion
Abnormal blood gases
Pursed lip breathing
Nasal flaring
Asymmetrical chest wall expansion
Somnolence
Cyanosis

Outcomes

Patient is free of respiratory distress.
Arterial blood·gases are within normal limit for patient.
Patient achieves optimal pulmonary function.

Documentation

Specify frequency.

Target date

Specify estimated date of completion.

Nursing interventions

Assess and document presence or absence of breath sounds, anterior and posterior, noting rales, rhonchi, wheezes, diminished breath sounds, and absence of breath sounds.

Review arterial blood gas results and correlate with clinical condition.

Report clinical changes and/or arterial blood gas results to physician.

Correlate all assessment data, document, and report any changes.

Instruct patient in relaxation techniques to improve breathing pattern.

Reassure patient during periods of respiratory distress.

Stay with patient during episodes of acute respiratory distress.

Maintain low flow oxygen by nasal cannula or mask.

Inform patient and family that smoking is prohibited in room.

Explain proper use of supportive equipment (O_2, suction, spirometer, IPPB).

Assess patient's lung sounds, respiratory rate, and production of sputum as indicators of effective use of supportive equipment.

Consult with physician regarding future need for arterial blood gas test and use of supportive equipment as indicated by a change in the patient's condition.

Other interventions specific to patient (specify).

Respiratory functions, Alteration in:
Mechanical ventilation

Related to: Disease process, Postoperative respiratory distress, Respiratory failure, Others specific to patient.

A condition in which the individual experiences an ineffective breathing pattern, necessitating the use of supportive respiratory equipment

Defining characteristics

Subjective

Complaining of severe breathing
  difficulty
Complaining of severe fatigue

Objective

Severe restlessness
Abnormal blood gases
Assymetric chest expansion
Absent or severely diminished breath
  sounds
Cyanosis
Apnea

Outcomes

Patient is free of respiratory distress.

Arterial blood gases are within normal limit for patient.

Patient demonstrates optimal breathing with assistance of mechanical ventilator.

Other outcomes specific to patient (specify).

Documentation
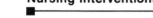

Specify frequency.

Target date

Specify estimated date of completion.

Nursing interventions

Assess and document need for percussion and/or supportive equipment.

Review results of arterial blood gases test and correlate with clinical condition.

Report clinical changes and/or results of arterial blood gases test to physician.

Assess and document synchronization of patient's breathing pattern with ventilator rate.

Observe and document bilateral chest expansion for patient on ventilator.

Correlate all assessment data, document, and report any changes.

Explain to patient and family the therapeutic function of the ventilator.

Inform patient of intended procedures before beginning them to lower anxiety and increase sense of control.

Provide care in a supportive manner, assessing patient for increased anxiety.

Consult with physician regarding need for sedation orders to help patient tolerate the ventilator.

Apply suction q ____. Be sure to hyperoxygenate with resuscitator bag prior to suctioning endotracheal tube or tracheostomy.

Confer with respiratory therapist to ensure the adequate functioning of the mechanical ventilator.

Other interventions specific to patient (specify).

Self-care deficit

Related to: Inability/limitation in: feeding, bathing/hygiene, dressing/grooming, toileting, Others specific to patient.

A condition in which an individual requires, or could require, assistance with the activities of daily living. Indicate area of limitation (feeding, bathing/hygiene, dressing/grooming, toileting) and functional level in each area of limitation (semidependent, moderately dependent, totally dependent). Definitions of functional levels appear in the table on page 85.

Defining characteristics

Subjective

Complaining of fatigue
Complaining of immobility
Complaining of lack of muscle strength
Complaining of pain
Demonstrating learned dependence
Demonstrating manipulative behavior toward staff and family
Demonstrating medication-induced lethargy
Expressing depression

Objective

Lack of muscle strength
Activity restrictions
Immobility due to casts/traction
Loss of limb, extremities
Paralysis
Confusion
Disorientation
Sensory deficit

Outcomes

Patient expresses acceptance of need for assistance with self care.
Patient is able to perform self care to optimal level.
Patient initiates plan to maintain personal hygiene.
Other outcomes specific to patient (specify).

Documentation

Specify frequency.

Target date

Specify estimated date of completion.

Nursing interventions

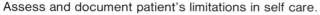

Assess and document patient's limitations in self care.

Encourage independence in performance of self care, assisting patient only as necessary.

Discuss limitations in self care with patient, and develop a self-care plan. Document agreed-upon self-care plan in nursing care plan.

Encourage patient to set own pace during self care.

Deliver care safely, patiently, and in a nonjudgmental manner.

Acknowledge and reinforce the patient's accomplishments.

Discuss the home environment with patient and family to help them plan for the self-care needs of the patient at home.

Offer pain medications prior to self care.

Other interventions specific to patient (specify).

Definitions and descriptors of functional level

	Semidependent	*Moderately dependent*	*Totally dependent*
Feeding	Nurse positions patient; gathers supplies; monitors eating.	Nurse cuts food; opens containers; positions patient; monitors and encourages eating.	Patient needs to be fed.
Bathing	Nurse provides all equipment; positions patient in bed/bathroom. Patient completes bath, except for back and feet.	Nurse supplies all equipment; positions patient; washes back, legs, perineum, and all other parts, as needed. Patient can assist.	Patient needs complete bath; cannot assist at all.
Oral hygiene	Nurse provides equipment; patient does task.	Nurse prepares brush; rinses patient's mouth; positions patient.	Nurse completes entire procedure.
Dressing/ grooming	Nurse gathers items for patient; may button, zip, or tie clothing; patient dresses self.	Nurse combs patient's hair; assists with dressing; buttons and zips clothing; ties shoes.	Patient needs to be dressed and cannot assist the nurse; nurse combs patient's hair.
Toileting	Patient can walk to bathroom/commode with assistance.	Nurse provides bedpan; positions patient on and off bedpan; places patient on bedside commode.	Patient is incontinent; nurse places patient on bedpan or commode.

Self-concept, Disturbance in

Related to: Body image disturbance, Personal identity disturbance, Role performance disruption, Self-esteem disturbances, Others specific to patient.

A condition in which an individual experiences, or could experience, all or any of the following:

Body image disturbance: Viewing oneself differently as a result of actual or perceived changes in body structure or function.

Personal identity disturbance: Disturbance in the perception of self, "Who am I?"

Role performance disruption: Inability to perform those functions and activities expected of a particular role in a given society.

Self-esteem disturbance: Lack of confidence in ability to accomplish what one wishes to accomplish.

Defining characteristics

Subjective

Showing reluctance to touch or look at affected body part
Stating "Why me?"
Expressing concern about ability to continue role performance
Expressing concern about significant other's response to body alteration
Expressing depression
Expressing anger
Expressing grief
Verbalizing despair
Family expressing concern about substance abuse
Family expressing concern about perceived change in familial relationships
Deferring self-care activities to others
Expressing difficulty in accepting positive reinforcement

Objective

Crying
Changes in appearance
Loss of body part
Apathy
Substance abuse
Labile affect

Outcomes

Patient verbalizes acceptance of self.
Patient verbalizes interest in appearance.
Patient demonstrates interest in appearance.
Patient verbalizes acceptance of alteration in appearance.
Patient demonstrates acceptance of alteration in appearance.
Patient maintains close personal relationships.
Patient verbalizes understanding of limitations.
Patient demonstrates ability to function within limitations.
Patient shows awareness of community resources.
Patient verbalizes willingness to change lifestyle.
Patient requests information appropriate to disease process.
Patient verbalizes awareness of change in role performance.
Patient identifies personal strengths that may enhance self-concept.
Other outcomes specific to patient (specify).

Documentation

Specify frequency.

Target date

Specify estimated date of completion.

(continued)

Nursing interventions
■───────────────────────────────

Assess and document evidence of disturbance in self-concept.

Encourage patient to verbalize consequences of physical and emotional changes that have influenced self-concept.

Encourage patient to maintain usual daily grooming routine.

Encourage patient to wear clothing to enhance physical and emotional self-esteem.

Help patient verbalize concerns about close personal relationships.

Encourage patient/family to ask questions about health concerns, treatments, progress, and prognosis.

Actively listen to patient/family and acknowledge reality of concerns, treatments, progress, and prognosis.

Encourage patient/family to air feelings and to grieve.

Provide care in a nonjudgmental manner, maintaining the patient's privacy and dignity.

Encourage patient to identify personal strengths that may enhance self-concept.

Help patient identify adaptive role performance behaviors.

Discuss with patient/family the impact of patient's change in role performance and the potential change in family members' role function.

Develop a plan of care with the patient that encourages patient/family participation and acknowledges limitations. Document plan of care in nursing care plan.

Help patient/family identify coping mechanisms related to: body image disturbance, personal identity disturbance, role performance disruption, and self-esteem disturbance.

Assess need for assistance from human support or social services department in planning approach and plan of care with patient/family.

Offer listing of community resources to patient/family.

Other interventions specific to patient (specify).

■───────────────────────────────

Sensory-perceptual alterations

Related to: Altered consciousness, Partial/total loss of hearing, Partial/ total loss of vision, Physiologic changes related to aging, Sensory overload, Others specific to patient.

A condition in which an individual experiences, or could experience, an alteration of sensory input because of the process of aging, excessive environmental stimuli, physiologic imbalance, and/or disorientation

Defining characteristics

Subjective

Expressing anxiety
Expressing fear
Expressing hallucinations
Solving problems ineffectively
Complaining of limited understanding
   of environment
Complaining of severe pain
Reporting substance abuse

Objective

Erratic sleep pattern
Limited concentration
Apathy
Abnormal/or lack of response
Abnormal laboratory results (electro-
   lytes, BUN, creatinine, ammonia)
Change in behavior pattern following
   medications
Regular intake of prescription or over-
   the-counter medications
Disorientation to person, place, or
   time
Labile affect
Hearing deficit
Decrease in visual acuity

Outcomes

Patient demonstrates ability to cope with stimuli.

Patient demonstrates accurate perception of environment.

Patient responds appropriately to environment.

Patient demonstrates the ability to adapt to physiologic changes.

Other outcomes specific to patient (specify).

Documentation

Specify frequency.

Target date

Specify estimated date of completion.

Nursing interventions

Assess and document patient's level of consciousness.

Assess and document patient's neurological status.

Assess and document changes in neurological status q ____.

Assess and document level of pain by patient's verbal and nonverbal cues.

Assess and document patient's ability to solve problems effectively, assisting as necessary.

Assess and document patient's concentration during conversation and teaching. Adjust teaching plan to accommodate patient's ability to concentrate.

Evaluate patient's perceptions of environmental stimuli.

Review laboratory results, medications administered, and input and output to monitor physiological homeostasis.

Identify factors that contribute to sensory-perceptual alteration.

Reduce or increase amount of stimuli to achieve appropriate sensory input. For example, speak clearly with low pitch to patients with hearing deficit; provide clock with large numbers for patient with decreased visual acuity.

Do not support hallucinations.

Evaluate sleep pattern as possible cause of altered perceptions.

Allow for flexibility in plan of care, involving patient in plan.

Encourage use of unimpaired senses.

Elicit information from patient about use of mind-altering substances. Document in nurse's notes.

Allow patient/family to verbalize anxiety.

When appropriate, reassure patient and family that sensory-perceptual deficit is temporary.

Other interventions specific to patient (specify).

Sexual dysfunction

Related to: Altered bladder control, Body image disturbance, Depression, Impotence, Loss of libido, Loss of sensation, Medications, Painful coitus, Others specific to patient.

A condition in which an individual experiences, or could experience, inadequacy, dissatisfaction, and/or incompatibility related to sexuality

Defining characteristics

Subjective

Expressing change in sexual relation-
ships
Expressing decrease in sexual desire
Expressing difficulty in sexual per-
formance
Expressing discontent with sexual
role, actual or perceived
Expressing fear of pregnancy
Expressing fear of venereal disease
Expressing limitations to sexual
activity imposed by disease,
therapy, or surgery
Expressing misinformation regarding
sexuality
Expressing sexual exploitation or
abuse
Expressing side-effects of medica-
tions

Outcomes

Patient verbalizes concerns about sexual dysfunction.
Patient acknowledges importance of discussing sexual issues with
partner.
Patient requests needed information about sexuality.
Other outcomes specific to patient (specify).

Documentation

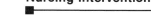

Specify frequency.

Target date

Specify estimated date of completion.

Nursing interventions

Discuss with patient the possibility of lack of interest in or desire for sexual activity.

Alert patient to possibility of decreased capacity for, or discomfort during, sexual activity.

The nurse should be aware of his or her own feelings about sexuality. If uncomfortable discussing sexual feelings, then request that someone else undertake patient teaching.

Confer with the physician about information needs expressed by patient so that teaching needs can be addressed.

Allow time and privacy to answer patient's questions concerning sexual dysfunction.

Encourage communication between patient and sexual partner.

Provide information on sexual dysfunction, being aware of verbal and nonverbal communication.

Provide written information, if available, that patient/family can use as a resource.

Other interventions specific to patient (specify).

Skin integrity, Impairment of

Related to: Draining wound, Long-term corticosteroid therapy, Immobility, Incontinence (stool/urine), Pressure ulcer, Stomal problems, Others specific to patient.

A condition in which the individual experiences, or could experience, an alteration in the skin surface that compromises it as a protective barrier

Defining characteristics

Subjective	Objective
Complaining of itching	Discolored skin
Complaining of pain, discomfort	Draining wound
Complaining of tenderness	Open skin lesion
	Poor skin turgor
	Presence of caustic liquid on skin (bile, wound drainage)
	Pressure area
	Pruritis
	Rash
	Thin skin

Outcomes

Patient is free of skin breakdown.

Patient is free of redness or excoriation in specified areas.

Patient has fewer incontinent episodes.

Patient is free of further skin breakdown.

Other outcomes specific to patient (specify).

Documentation

Specify frequency.

Target date

Specify estimated date of completion.

Nursing interventions

Assess and document condition of skin over bony prominences for breakdown.

Assess and document presence/absence of redness, excoriation, pain, itching, and tenderness.

Assess and document need for indwelling or condom catheter.

Check for incontinence q _____.

Cleanse perianal area with water and nondrying soap after incontinence.

Put patient on bedpan q _____.

Take patient to bathroom q _____.

Give circular massage over bony prominences q _____.

Turn and reposition patient q _____.

If protective clothing is used to contain incontinence, change it frequently.

Use protective measures, such as stomahesive, egg crate mattress, foam protectors.

Provide foods high in proteins, minerals, and vitamins.

Administer care for decubitus ulcer.

Instruct patient to avoid extremes in temperature (heating pad, ice) over affected area.

Other interventions specific to patient (specify).

Sleep pattern disturbance

Related to: Medication use, Sleep deprivation, Others specific to patient.

A condition in which the individual experiences, or could experience, a disruption in the amount and/or quality of sleep

Defining characteristics

Subjective

Complaining of difficulty in falling asleep
Complaining of fatigue
Complaining of irritability
Complaining of mood alterations
Complaining of wakefulness

Objective

Frequent daytime napping
Frequent yawning
Constant coughing
Decreased attention span
Nocturia
Regular use of sedative/hypnotic medications
Regular use of medications that can change sleep patterns

Outcomes

Patient reports adequate rest.

Patient uses sleeping aids appropriately.

Other outcomes specific to patient (specify).

Documentation

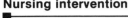

Specify frequency.

Target date

Specify estimated date of completion.

Nursing interventions

Assess and document patient's sleeping pattern and need for sleeping aids.

Help patient identify sleeping pattern while in hospital.

Help patient identify possible underlying causes of sleeplessness, such as fear, unresolved problems, and conflicts.

Provide comfort measures at hour of sleep and nap time.

Provide quiet, peaceful environment, minimizing interruptions.

Discuss usual sleep aids, e.g., back rub, warm milk, soft music, with patient.

Plan activities to allow time for sleep/rest.

Offer sleep medications, if appropriate, avoiding long-term nightly use.

Confer with physician regarding need to revise medication regimen when nonhypnotic medications interfere with sleep pattern.

Encourage patient to verbalize need for sleep/rest.

Find a compatible roommate for the patient, if possible.

Avoid unnecessary procedures during sleep period.

Avoid loud noises and use of overhead lights during nighttime sleep.

Limit visiting during rest periods.

Evaluate need for sleep medication, taking into account necessary activities during nighttime.

Inform patient that irritability and mood alterations are commonly a consequence of sleep deprivation.

Other interventions specific to patient (specify).

Social isolation

Related to: Chemical dependency, Chronologic age, Medical condition, Physical handicap, Sexual preference, Others specific to patient.

A condition in which an individual experiences, or could experience, an inability to establish and/or maintain relationships with others, despite a desire for socialization

Defining characteristics

Subjective

Verbalizing inadequacy in establishing or maintaining relationship with others
Verbalizing loneliness
Verbalizing fear of others
Expressing negative self-image
Expressing anger

Objective

Demonstrated inability to interact with others
Indecisiveness
Restlessness
Sleep disturbance
Withdrawal

Outcomes

Patient verbalizes a need for social contact with others.

Patient identifies behaviors that produce social isolation.

Patient demonstrates acceptance of own personal characteristics, such as age, sexual preference, or physical disability, that are perceived to contribute to social isolation.

Patient verbalizes behaviors that may increase social interaction.

Other outcomes specific to patient (specify).

Documentation

Specify frequency.

Target date

Specify estimated date of completion.

Nursing interventions

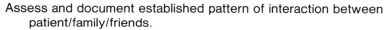

Assess and document established pattern of interaction between patient/family/friends.

Assess and document cues that may help the patient identify his or her feelings of isolation.

Encourage patient to verbalize feelings of social isolation.

Establish, implement, and evaluate a plan to increase the patient's interaction with others.

Reinforce efforts by patient/family/friends to establish interaction.

Confer with social services about patient's need to increase social interaction.

Provide information on community resources that will promote increased social interaction after discharge.

Assist patient in decision-making process by limiting choices that produce anxiety. Give positive reinforcement for decision making.

Provide diversion during daylight hours to promote socialization and to establish routine sleeping patterns at night.

Other interventions specific to patient (specify).

Spiritual distress

Related to: Discrepancy between spiritual beliefs and prescribed treatment, Disruption in spiritual practices, Test of spiritual beliefs, Others specific to patient.

A condition in which an individual experiences, or could experience, a disruption in a belief and value system that is a usual source of security and strength for the patient

Defining characteristics

Subjective

Abandoning usual belief system
Asking "Why did this happen to me?"
Expressing concern about non-adherence to dietary laws
Expressing frustration about non-participation in usual spiritual practices
Expressing guilt
Requesting spiritual counseling
Requesting objects associated with worship
Questioning existence or fairness of the supreme being

Objective

Withdrawal
Disruption in sleep pattern
Crying
Refusal to accept visits from priest, minister, rabbi, etc.

Outcomes

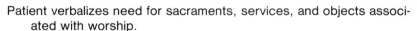

Patient verbalizes need for sacraments, services, and objects associated with worship.
Patient demonstrates comfort with spiritual observances.
Patient attends religious services in the hospital, if desired.
Patient verbalizes concerns about inability to adhere to dietary laws.
Patient expresses reconciliation with usual belief system.
Other outcomes specific to patient (specify).

Documentation

Specify frequency.

Target date

Specify estimated date of completion.

Nursing interventions

Assess and document patient's religious and spiritual needs when obtaining nursing history upon admission.

Communicate acceptance of and respect for patient's religious beliefs by involving the patient in the planning of care.

Provide privacy and time for patient to observe religious practices.

Contact denominational representative in community and/or hospital upon request of patient/family.

If patient indicates a dietary restriction (e.g., kosher food, vegetarian diet, pork-free diet), consult with the dietitian to evaluate patient's dietary needs.

Encourage patient's family or friends to bring special food.

Provide religious reading material upon patient's request.

Acknowledge limitations that hospitalization imposes on religious observances.

Recognize nurse's own limitations in understanding patient's religious beliefs, communicating in a nonjudgmental manner.

Other interventions specific to patient (specify).

Thought process, Alteration in

Related to: Impaired perception of reality, Psychological changes related to aging, Others specific to patient.

A condition in which an individual experiences, or could experience, an inability to comprehend, solve problems, or perceive reality

Defining characteristics

Subjective

Complaining of fearful thoughts
Complaining of hallucinations
Complaining of irritability
Complaining of memory loss

Objective

Inappropriate affect or responses
Restlessness
Verbalization of incomplete thoughts
Inaccurate interpretation of environ-
    mental stimuli
Disorientation
Distraction
Inability to solve problems
Regressive behavior
Preoccupation with self

Outcomes

Patient is oriented to person.

Patient is oriented to place.

Patient is oriented to time.

Patient achieves preillness mental status.

Patient achieves improved mental status.

Patient is free from injury.

Patient demonstrates improved ability to solve problems.

Patient verbalizes no hallucinations or delusions.

Patient verbalizes appropriate responses.

Patient demonstrates appropriate behavior.

Other outcomes specific to patient (specify).

Documentation

Specify frequency.

Target date

Specify estimated date of completion.

Nursing interventions

Assess and document patient's orientation to person, place, and time.

Reorient to person, place, and time q ____.

Correlate initial baseline assessment of mental status with present assessment.

Assist patient with ambulation and activities of daily living as necessary.

Assist patient in solving problems.

Encourage patient to participate in plan of care.

Use environmental stimuli, such as a calendar, clock, and pictures.

Provide and document a safe patient environment.

Apply soft restraints, as necessary.

Provide diversion to assist with reorientation.

Explain to patient/family the relationship between confusion and patient's diagnosis.

Explain all procedures to patient/family.

Provide support to patient/family during patient's periods of disorientation.

Provide positive feedback and reinforcement of appropriate behavior.

Instruct family/significant other to reorient patient, as needed.

Do not support patient's hallucinations.

Other interventions specific to patient (specify).

Tissue perfusion, Alteration in: *Peripheral*

Related to: Impaired circulation, Others specific to patient.

A condition in which an individual experiences, or could experience, inadequate blood supply through the vascular and/or lymphatic system

Defining characteristics

Subjective

Complaining of loss of sensation
Complaining of numbness
Complaining of pain
Complaining of pain in lower extremities when walking
Complaining of tingling sensations

Objective

Absence/decrease of peripheral pulses
Cool skin
Cyanosis
Flushed appearance of skin
Edema
Necrotic tissue
Skin lesions

Outcomes

Patient has palpable peripheral pulses.

Patient's affected limb is pink, not red or cyanotic, when in dependent position.

Patient's capillary refill is within normal limits or less than 3 seconds.

Patient reports decreased numbness and tingling in extremity.

Patient reports increased sensation in extremity.

Patient's edema decreases.

Patient's lesions begin to heal.

Skin temperature of extremity is within normal limits for patient.

Patient can move affected extremtity.

Patient reports adequate pain relief.

Other outcomes specific to patient (specify).

Documentation

Specify frequency.

Target date

Specify estimated date of completion.

Nursing interventions

Assess and document presence or absence of mottling in limb to assess capillary refill q _____.

Assess and document rate, rhythm, and volume of peripheral pulses to assess circulation in limb.

Assess and document for capillary filling and skin temperature q _____.

Assess and document presence of edema on scale from 1+ to 4+.

Assess and document effects of medications on tissue perfusion.

Assess and document need for antiembolus hose.

Correlate initial assessment with daily assessment, noting any increase or decrease of circulation in extremities.

Instruct patient to inform nurse of presence or absence of numbness or tingling in extremity.

Offer pain medications q _____ and document response.

Notify physician if pain is unrelieved.

Elevate extremity above heart to improve venous blood flow.

Place extremity in dependent position q _____ to improve arterial blood flow.

Avoid chemical, mechanical, or thermal trauma to involved extremity.

Discourage leg crossing or sitting for long periods to avoid compromising circulation to extremities.

Use foot cradle to avoid pressure of covers on extremities.

Discourage smoking and use of stimulants.

Encourage active/passive range-of-motion exercises with affected extremities q _____.

Provide meticulous hygiene to extremities.

Instruct patient to avoid applying extremes of temperature to extremities.

Instruct patient in importance of exercise program, correct diet, and adherence to medication regimen.

Consult with dietitian for diet instruction.

Other interventions specific to patient (specify).

Urinary elimination,
Alteration in pattern

Related to: Specific to patient.

A condition in which an individual experiences, or could experience, a disruption of usual urinary elimination pattern

Defining characteristics

Subjective

Complaining of bladder spasms
Complaining of frequency
Complaining of hesitancy
Complaining of pain during urination
Complaining of urgency
Complaining of urinary retention

Objective

Dribbling
Hematuria
Incontinence
Urinary retention

Outcomes

Patient reports lessening of painful urination.

Patient has fewer incontinent episodes.

Patient passes clear or clearing urine.

Patient reports decreased bladder spasms.

Patient demonstrates decreasing retention by voiding at least ____ cc each time he or she urinates.

Patient will demonstrate Foley catheter output at least ____ cc/hour.

Other outcomes specific to patient (specify).

Documentation
▬————————————————————————————————

Specify frequency.

Target date
▬————————————————————————————————

Specify estimated date of completion.

Nursing interventions
▬————————————————————————————————

Assess and document patient's usual urinary elimination pattern on admission.

Assess and document color and consistency of urine.

Assess and document presence or absence of bladder distention by palpation.

Assess and document for adequate Foley catheter output of at least _____ cc/hour.

Record time and amount of output q _____.

Encourage oral intake of fluids, unless contraindicated.

Provide privacy during urination.

Reassure patient, if appropriate, that dysuria is usually temporary.

Medicate prior to elimination to reduce pain during urination.

Establish voiding routine for patient by offering urinal or bedpan at regular intervals.

Implement techniques that may precipitate urination, such as: running water in sink, running warm water over patient's hands, having patient inhale oil of peppermint, providing warm blanket to pelvis.

Assist patient to bathroom at bedtime and encourage voiding to reduce urgency during the night.

Assist patient with use of urinal or bedpan at bedtime to reduce urgency during the night.

Consult with physician regarding need for sitz baths, pain medications, antispasmodics.

Consult with physician regarding order for catheter irrigation, if needed.

Encourage patient to stand or sit when voiding.

Answer patient call light in a timely manner.

Provide care in a nonjudgmental manner, maintaining the patient's privacy and dignity.

Use protective garments to protect skin of incontinent patient.

Other interventions specific to patient (specify).

▬————————————————————————————————

Violence, Potential for

Related to: Impaired behavior patterns, Others specific to patient.

A condition in which an individual displays, or could display, verbal and/or physical abusive behavior toward self or others

Defining characteristics

Subjective	*Objective*
Expressing delusions	Clenched fists
Expressing hallucinations	Aggressive behavior
Expressing irritability	Agitation
Expressing suspicions of people	Hostile language
Expressing suspicions of environment	Pacing
Expressing anxiety	Reported/known history of abusive behavior
	Reported/known history of substance abuse
	Withdrawal

Outcomes

Patient verbalizes anger.

Patient reports increasing ability to control anger.

Patient/family acknowledge role of anger in disease process.

Patient identifies effective ways to express anger in a nondestructive manner.

Patient demonstrates ability to control aggressive behavior toward self and others.

Other outcomes specific to patient (specify).

Documentation
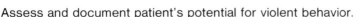

Specify frequency.

Target date

Specify estimated date of completion.

Nursing interventions

Assess and document patient's potential for violent behavior.

Assess and document patient's potential for suicide.

Encourage patient to verbalize anger.

Set limits on patient's behavior and document limits in nurse's notes.

Provide a safe environment by removing items that may endanger patient and others.

Discuss with patient/family the role of anger in disease process.

Help patient to control anger by anticipating events that may precipitate aggressive episodes.

Provide positive feedback when patient adheres to behavior limits.

Provide care in a calm, efficient manner, offering reassurance and support.

Confer with human support/social services to devise a plan of care.

Use appropriate restraining measures when necessary to prevent injury to patient and others.

Encourage the use of positive coping mechanisms, such as relaxation techniques, exercise, etc.

Other interventions specific to patient (specify).

Nursing Diagnoses Guide
to Medical and Surgical Conditions

Medical Conditions

Abdominal pain

Activity intolerance
Related to: Pain, Weakness/fatigue

Anxiety
Related to: Specific to patient

Bowel elimination, Alteration in: Constipation
Related to: Decreased activity, Decreased fluid intake, Dietary changes, Disease process

Bowel elimination, Alteration in: Diarrhea
Related to: Dietary changes, Disease process, Impaction

Comfort, Alteration in
Related to: Pain (acute)

Coping, Ineffective individual
Related to: Anxiety

Fear
Related to: Disease process, Hospitalization, Invasive medical procedure, Real or imagined threat to well-being

Fluid volume, Alteration in: Excess
Related to: Ascites

Fluid volume deficit
Related to: Abnormal fluid loss, Decreased fluid intake

Knowledge deficit
Related to: Limited understanding of prescribed treatment

Nutrition, Alteration in: Less than body requirements
Related to: Loss of appetite, Nausea and vomiting

Respiratory functions, Alteration in: Breathing pattern, ineffective
Related to: Abdominal distention

Self-care deficit
Related to: Inability/limitations in: bathing, toileting

Sleep pattern disturbance
Related to: Sleep deprivation

Angina, coronary insufficiency

Activity intolerance
Related to: Anxiety, Arrhythmias, Impaired gas exchange, Pain, Weakness and fatigue

Anxiety
Related to: Specific to patient

Cardiac output, Alteration in: Decreased
Related to: Arrhythmia, Drug intolerance, Stress on heart's function

Comfort, Alteration in
Related to: Bed rest, Pain (acute)

Coping, Ineffective individual
Related to: Anger, Anxiety, Denial, Dependent behavior, Depression

Family process, Alteration in
Related to: Care of elderly family member, Complex therapies, Hospitalization, Illness of family member

Fear
Related to: Disease process, Hospitalization, Invasive medical procedures, Powerlessness, Real or imagined threat to well-being

Fluid volume, Alteration in: Excess
Related to: Specific to patient

Knowledge deficit
Related to: Limited understanding of prescribed treatment

Mobility, Impaired physical
Related to: Decreased strength and
endurance

Noncompliance
Related to: Negative consequence of
treatment regimen, Dysfunctional relationship with health care providers

**Nutrition, Alteration in: Less than
body requirements**
Related to: Inadequate nutrition

**Respiratory functions, Alteration in:
Gas exchange, impaired**
Related to: Specific to patient

Self-care deficit
Related to: Inability/limitations in:
feeding, bathing/hygiene, dressing/
grooming, toileting

Self-concept, Disturbance in
Related to: Body image, Personal
identity, Role-performance, Self-
esteem

Sexual dysfunction
Related to: Body image, Depression,
Impotence

Sleep pattern disturbance
Related to: Sleep deprivation

Thought process, Alteration in
Related to: Impaired perception of
reality

Autoimmune disorders

*Includes, but is not limited to: Ac-
quired Immune Deficiency Syndrome
(AIDS); Rheumatoid Arthritis; Systemic
Lupus Erythematosus; Scleroderma;
Vasculitis. See Nursing Diagnosis list
for Infection.*

Activity intolerance
Related to: Anxiety, Pain, Weakness/
fatigue

Anxiety
Related to: Specific to patient

Fear
Related to: Disease process, Hospitalization, Invasive medical procedures, Powerlessness, Real or
imagined threat to well-being

**Bowel elimination, Alteration in:
Constipation**
Related to: Decreased activity,
Decreased fluid intake, Dietary
changes, Medications

**Bowel elimination, Alteration in:
Diarrhea**
Related to: Medication, Stress

Comfort, Alteration in
Related to: Pain (acute), Pain
(chronic)

Coping, Ineffective individual
Related to: Anger, Anxiety, Denial,
Dependent behavior, Depression

Family process, Alteration in
Related to: Care of elderly family
member, Change in family roles, Complex therapies, Hospitalization, Illness
of family member

Grieving
Related to: Actual or perceived loss,
Anticipated loss

Health maintenance, Alterations in
Related to: Health beliefs

**Home maintenance management,
Impaired**
Related to: Home environment ob-
stacles, Inadequate support system,
Insufficient family organization or
planning

Injury, Potential for
Related to: Motor deficit, Sensory
deficit

Knowledge deficit
Related to: Limited understanding of
disease process, Limited understanding of prescribed treatment

Autoimmune disorders *(continued)*

Mobility, Impaired physical
Related to: Decreased strength and endurance, Musculoskeletal impairment

Noncompliance
Related to: Dysfunctional relationship with health care providers, Negative consequence of treatment regimen, Negative perception of treatment regimen

Nutrition, Alteration in: Less than body requirements
Related to: High metabolic states, Inadequate nutrition, Loss of appetite, Nausea and vomiting

Oral mucous membranes, Alteration in
Related to: Stomatitis

Powerlessness
Related to: Disease process, Hospitalization

Respiratory functions, Alteration in: Airway clearance, ineffective; Breathing pattern, ineffective; Gas exchange, impaired
Related to: Disease process

Self-care deficit
Related to: Inability/limitations in: feeding, bathing/hygiene, dressing/ grooming, toileting

Self-concept, Disturbance in: Altered body image
Related to: Body image, Personal identity, Role performance, Self-esteem

Sensory-perceptual alterations
Related to: Physiologic changes related to aging, Sensory overload

Sexual dysfunction
Related to: Body image disturbance, Depression, Impotence, Medications, Physiologic limitations

Skin integrity, Impairment of
Related to: Altered sensation, Long-term steroid therapy, Immobility

Social isolation
Related to: Chronologic age, Medical condition, Physical handicaps, Sexual preference

Thought process, Alteration in
Related to: Psychological changes related to aging

Tissue perfusion, Alteration in
Related to: Impaired circulation

Blood dyscrasias
■───────────────────────

Includes, but not limited to: Aplastic Anemia; Pernicious Anemia; Sickle Cell Anemia. See Nursing Diagnosis list for Infection.

Activity Intolerance
Related to: Anxiety, Impaired gas exchange, Pain, Weakness/ fatigue

Anxiety
Related to: Specific to patient

Bowel elimination, Alteration in: Constipation
Related to: Decreased activity, Decreased fluid intake, Dietary changes, Disease process, Medications

Comfort, Alteration in
Related to: Bed rest, Pain (acute), Pain (chronic)

Coping, Ineffective individual
Related to: Anger, Anxiety, Denial, Dependent behavior, Depression

Family process, Alteration in
Related to: Care of elderly family member, Change in family roles, Complex therapies, Hospitalization, Illness of family member

Fear
Related to: Disease process, Hospitalization, Invasive medical procedures, Powerlessness, Real or imagined threat to well-being

Knowledge deficit
Related to: Limited understanding of disease process, Limited understanding of prescribed treatment

Mobility, Impaired physical
Related to: Decreased strength and endurance, Musculoskeletal impairment

Nutrition, Alteration in: Less than body requirements
Related to: High metabolic states, Inadequate nutrition, Loss of appetite, Nausea and vomiting

Oral mucous membranes, Alteration in
Related to: Stomatitis

Respiratory functions, Alteration in: Breathing pattern, ineffective
Related to: Disease process

Self-care deficit
Related to: Inability/limitation in: bathing/hygiene, dressing/grooming, toileting

Sleep pattern disturbance
Related to: Medications, Sleep deprivation

Burns

Activity intolerance
Related to: Pain

Anxiety
Related to: Specific to patient

Bowel elimination, Alteration in: Constipation
Related to: Decreased activity, Medications

Cardiac output, Alteration in: Decreased
Related to: Stress on heart's function

Comfort, Alteration in
Related to: Pain (acute)

Coping, Ineffective individual
Related to: Anger, Anxiety, Denial, Dependent behavior, Depression

Diversional activity deficit
Related to: Boredom

Family process, Alteration in
Related to: Complex therapies, Hospitalization

Fear
Related to: Hospitalization, Invasive medical procedures, Powerlessness, Real or imagined threat to well-being

Fluid volume, Alteration in: Excess
Related to: Specific to patient

Fluid volume deficit
Related to: Abnormal fluid loss, Decreased fluid intake

Injury, Potential for
Related to: Sensory deficit

Knowledge deficit
Related to: Limited understanding of prescribed treatment

Mobility, Impaired physical
Related to: Decreased strength and endurance, Musculoskeletal impairment

Noncompliance
Related to: Dysfunctional relationship with health care providers, Negative consequence of treatment regimen

Burns *(continued)*

Nutrition, Alteration in: Less than body requirements
Related to: Difficulty swallowing, High metabolic requirements, Inadequate nutrition, Loss of appetite, Nausea and vomiting

Powerlessness
Related to: Hospitalization

Self-care deficit
Related to: Inability/limitations in: feeding, bathing/hygiene, dressing/ grooming, toileting

Self-concept, Disturbance in
Related to: Body image, Personal identity, Role performance, Self- esteem

Sensory-perceptual alterations
Related to: Sensory overload

Skin integrity, Impairment of
Related to: Altered sensation, Immo- bility

Sleep pattern disturbance
Related to: Sleep deprivation

Urinary elimination, Alteration in pattern
Related to: Specific to patient

Cancer

Anxiety
Related to: Specific to patient

Bowel elimination, Alteration in: Constipation
Related to: Decreased activity, Dietary changes, Medications, Painful defecation

Bowel elimination, Alteration in: Diarrhea
Related to: Dietary changes, Disease process, Impaction, Medication, Stress

Bowel elimination, Alteration in: Incontinence
Related to: Disease process, Loss of sphincter control

Comfort, Alteration in
Related to: Bed rest, Pain

Coping, Ineffective individual
Related to: Anger, Anxiety, Depen- dent behavior, Depression

Family process, Alteration in
Related to: Care of elderly family member, Change in family roles, Com- plex therapies, Hospitalization, Illness of family member

Fear
Related to: Disease process, Hos- pitalization, Invasive medical pro- cedures, Powerlessness, Real or imagined threat to well-being, Surgical procedure

Fluid volume, Alteration in: Excess
Related to: Ascites

Fluid volume deficit
Related to: Abnormal fluid loss, De- creased fluid intake

Grieving
Related to: Actual or perceived loss, Anticipated loss

Home maintenance management, Impaired
Related to: Disease of family member other than patient, Home environment obstacles, Inadequate support sys- tem, Insufficient family organization or planning

Knowledge deficit
Related to: Limited understanding of prescribed treatment

Mobility, Impaired physical
Related to: Decreased strength and endurance

Noncompliance
Related to: Negative consequence of treatment regimen, Dysfunctional relationship with health care providers

Nutrition, Alteration in: Less than body requirements
Related to: Difficulty swallowing, Inadequate nutrition, Loss of appetite, Nausea and vomiting

Oral mucous membranes, Alteration in
Related to: Stomatitis

Powerlessness
Related to: Hospitalization

Respiratory functions, Alteration in: Airway clearance, ineffective; Breathing pattern, ineffective; Gas exchange, impaired
Depending on location. Related to: Specific to patient.

Self-care deficit
Related to: Inability/limitations in: feeding, bathing/hygiene, dressing/grooming, toileting

Self-concept, Disturbance in
Related to: Body image, Personal identity, Role performance, Self-esteem

Sensory-perceptual alterations
Related to: Altered consciousness, Sensory overload, Physiologic changes related to aging

Sexual dysfunction
Related to: Altered bladder control, Depression, Impotence, Physiological limitations

Skin integrity, Impairment of
Related to: Draining wound, Immobility, Pressure ulcer, Stomal problems

Sleep pattern disturbance
Related to: Sleep deprivation

Social isolation
Related to: Chronologic age, Medical condition

Spiritual distress
Related to: Discrepancy between spiritual beliefs and prescribed treatment, Disruption in spiritual practices, Test of spiritual beliefs

Thought process, Alteration in
Related to: Impaired perception of reality

Urinary elimination, Alteration in pattern
Depending on location. Related to: Specific to patient.

Cerebrovascular accident

Activity intolerance
Related to: Weakness and fatigue

Anxiety
Related to: Specific to patient

Bowel elimination, Alteration in: Constipation
Related to: Decreased activity, Medications

Bowel elimination, Alteration in: Diarrhea
Related to: Impaction

Bowel elimination, Alteration in: Incontinence
Related to: Loss of sphincter control

Coping, Ineffective individual
Related to: Anger, Denial, Depression

Communication, Impaired verbal
Related to: Aphasia

Diversional activity deficit
Related to: Boredom

Family process, Alteration in
Related to: Change in family roles, Hospitalization

Cerebrovascular accident *(continued)*

Fear
Related to: Disease process, Hospitalization, Invasive medical procedures, Powerlessness, Real or imagined threat to well-being

Fluid volume deficit
Related to: Abnormal fluid loss, Decreased fluid intake

Health maintenance, Alterations in
Related to: Health beliefs

Home maintenance management, Impaired
Related to: Home environment obstacles, Inadequate support system

Injury, Potential for
Related to: Motor deficit, Sensory deficit

Knowledge deficit
Related to: Limited understanding of prescribed treatment

Mobility, Impaired physical
Related to: Decreased strength and endurance, Musculoskeletal impairment, Neuromuscular impairment

Nutrition, Alteration in: Less than body requirements
Related to: Difficulty swallowing, Inadequate nutrition, Loss of appetite, Nausea and vomiting

Powerlessness
Related to: Hospitalization

Self-care deficit
Related to: Inability/limitations in: bathing/hygiene, dressing/grooming, toileting

Self-concept, Disturbance in
Related to: Body image, Role performance, Self-esteem

Sensory-perceptual alterations
Related to: Altered consciousness

Skin integrity, Impairment of
Related to: Immobility, Incontinence (stool/urine), Pressure ulcer

Sleep pattern disturbance
Related to: Sleep deprivation

Spiritual distress
Related to: Discrepancy between spiritual beliefs and prescribed treatment, Disruption in spiritual practices

Thought process, Alteration in
Related to: Impaired perception of reality

Urinary elimination, Alteration in pattern
Related to: Specific to patient

Violence, Potential for
Related to: Impaired behavior patterns

Chest injury

Activity intolerance
Related to: Anxiety, Weakness and fatigue

Anxiety
Related to: Specific to patient

Comfort, Alteration in
Related to: Pain

Coping, Ineffective individual
Related to: Anxiety

Fear
Related to: Hospitalization, Invasive medical procedures, Powerlessness, Real or imagined threat to well-being

Fluid volume deficit
Related to: Abnormal fluid loss

Mobility, Impaired physical
Related to: Musculoskeletal impairment

Respiratory functions, Alteration in: Breathing pattern, ineffective; Gas exchange, impaired
Related to: Specific to patient

Self-care deficit
Related to: Inability/limitations in: feeding, bathing/hygiene, dressing/ grooming, toileting

Self-concept, Disturbance in
Related to: Body image

Sleep pattern disturbance
Related to: Sleep deprivation

Chronic obstructive pulmonary disease

■────────────────

Includes, but is not limited to: Asthma; Bronchitis; Emphysema.

Activity intolerance
Related to: Arrhythmias, Impaired gas exchange, Weakness and fatigue

Anxiety
Related to: Specific to patient

Cardiac output, Alteration in: Decreased
Related to: Arrhythmias, Stress on heart's function, Drug intolerance

Coping, Ineffective individual
Related to: Anger, Anxiety, Dependent behavior, Depression

Family process, Alteration in
Related to: Care of elderly family member, Hospitalization

Fear
Related to: Disease process, Hospitalization, Powerlessness, Real or imagined threat to well-being

Fluid volume deficit
Related to: Abnormal fluid loss, Decreased fluid intake

Health maintenance, Alterations in
Related to: Health beliefs

Home maintenance management, Impaired
Related to: Disease of family member other than patient, Home environment obstacles, Inadequate support system, Insufficient family organization or planning

Knowledge deficit
Related to: Limited understanding of prescribed treatment

Mobility, Impaired physical
Related to: Decreased strength and endurance

Noncompliance
Related to: Negative consequence of treatment regimen, Dysfunctional relationship with health care providers

Nutrition, Alteration in: Less than body requirements
Related to: Inadequate nutrition, Loss of appetite, Nausea and vomiting

Powerlessness
Related to: Hospitalization

Respiratory functions, Alteration in: Airway clearance, ineffective; Breathing pattern, ineffective; Gas exchange, impaired; Mechanical ventilation
Related to: Specific to patient

Self-care deficit
Related to: Inability/limitations in: feeding, bathing/hygiene, dressing/ grooming, toileting

Self-concept, Disturbance in
Related to: Body image, Personal identity, Role performance, Self-esteem

Skin integrity, Impairment of
Related to: Immobility

Sleep pattern disturbance
Related to: Sleep deprivation

Congestive heart failure

Activity intolerance
Related to: Weakness/fatigue

Anxiety
Related to: Specific to patient

Cardiac output, Alteration in: Decreased
Related to: Arrhythmia, Stress on heart's function

Coping, Ineffective individual
Related to: Anxiety, Denial, Dependent behavior, Depression

Fear
Related to: Disease process, Hospitalization, Invasive medical procedures, Real or imagined threat to well-being

Fluid volume, Alteration in: Excess
Related to: Specific to patient

Fluid volume deficit
Related to: Decreased fluid intake

Health maintenance, Alterations in
Related to: Health beliefs

Home maintenance management, Impaired
Related to: Disease of family member other than patient, Home environment obstacles, Inadequate support system, Insufficient family organization or planning

Knowledge deficit
Related to: Limited understanding of prescribed treatment

Mobility, Impaired physical
Related to: Decreased strength and endurance

Noncompliance
Related to: Negative consequence of treatment regimen

Nutrition, Alteration in: Less than body requirements
Related to: Difficulty swallowing, Inadequate nutrition, Loss of appetite, Nausea and vomiting

Respiratory functions, Alteration in: Airway clearance, ineffective; Breathing pattern, ineffective; Gas exchange, impaired
Related to: Specific to patient

Self-care deficit
Related to: Inability/limitations in: feeding, bathing/hygiene, dressing/grooming, toileting

Self-concept, Disturbance in:
Related to: Role performance

Sensory-perceptual alterations
Related to: Physiologic changes related to aging, Sensory overload

Skin integrity, Impairment of
Related to: Immobility, Incontinence (stool/urine), Pressure ulcer

Sleep pattern disturbance
Related to: Sleep deprivation

Thought process, Alteration in
Related to: Impaired perception of reality

Tissue perfusion, Alteration in
Related to: Impaired circulation

Elderly patient

Activity intolerance
Related to: Arrhythmias, Impaired gas exchange, Pain, Weakness/fatigue

Anxiety
Related to: Specific to patient

Bowel elimination, Alteration in: Constipation
Related to: Aging process, Decreased activity, Dietary changes, Medications, Painful defecation

Bowel elimination, Alteration in: Diarrhea
Related to: Dietary changes, Disease process, Impaction, Medication, Stress

Bowel elimination, Alteration in: Incontinence
Related to: Decreased awareness of need to defecate, Disease process, Loss of sphincter control

Cardiac output, Alteration in
Related to: Arrhythmia, Drug intolerance, Stress on heart's function

Coping, Ineffective individual
Related to: Anger, Anxiety, Denial, Dependent behavior, Depression

Family process, Alteration in
Related to: Care of elderly family member, Change in family roles, Hospitalization

Fear
Related to: Disease process, Hospitalization, Invasive medical procedures, Powerlessness, Real or imagined threat to well-being, Surgical procedure

Fluid volume deficit
Related to: Abnormal fluid loss, Decreased fluid intake

Health maintenance, Alterations in
Related to: Health beliefs

Home maintenance management, Impaired
Related to: Disease of family member other than patient, Home environment obstacles, Inadequate support system, Insufficient family organization or planning

Injury, Potential for
Related to: Hypotension, Motor deficit, Sensory deficit, Substance intoxication, Psychomotor hyperactivity

Knowledge deficit
Related to: Limited understanding of disease process, Limited understanding of prescribed treatment

Mobility, Impaired physical
Related to: Decreased strength and endurance, Musculoskeletal impairment, Neuromuscular impairment

Noncompliance
Related to: Negative consequence of treatment regimen, Dysfunctional relationship with health care providers

Nutrition, Alteration in: Less than body requirements
Related to: Difficulty swallowing, Inadequate nutrition, Loss of appetite, Nausea and vomiting

Powerlessness
Related to: Hospitalization

Respiratory functions, Alteration in: Breathing pattern, ineffective; Gas exchange, impaired
Related to: Specific to patient

Self-care deficit
Related to: Inability/limitations in: feeding, bathing/hygiene, dressing/grooming, toileting

Self-concept, Disturbance in
Related to: Body image, Personal identity, Role performance, Self-esteem

Sensory-perceptual alterations
Related to: Altered consciousness, Partial/total loss of hearing, Partial/total loss of vision, Physiologic changes related to aging, Sensory overload

Sexual dysfunction
Related to: Altered bladder control, Body image, Depression, Impotence, Medications, Physiological limitations

Elderly patient *(continued)*

Skin integrity, Impairment of
Related to: Altered sensation, Immobility, Incontinence (stool, urine), Pressure ulcer

Sleep pattern disturbance
Related to: Medications, Sleep deprivation

Spiritual distress
Related to: Discrepancy between spiritual beliefs and prescribed treatment, Disruption in spiritual practices, Test of spiritual beliefs

Social isolation
Related to: Chronologic age, Medical condition, Physical handicaps

Thought process, Alteration in
Related to: Impaired perception of reality

Tissue perfusion, Alteration in
Related to: Impaired circulation

Urinary elimination, Alteration in pattern
Related to: Specific to patient

Endocrine disorders
■

Includes, but not limited to: Cushing's Disease; Diabetes Mellitus; Hyperthyroidism; Hypoglycemia; Hypothyroidism; Pancreatic Tumors.

Anxiety
Related to: Specific to patient

Coping, Ineffective individual
Related to: Anger, Anxiety, Denial, Dependent behavior, Depression

Family process, Alteration in
Related to: Care of elderly family member, Change in family roles, Complex therapies, Hospitalization, Illness of family member

Fear
Related to: Disease process, Hospitalization, Invasive medical procedures, Powerlessness, Real or imagined threat to well-being

Fluid volume deficit
Related to: Abnormal fluid loss, Decreased fluid intake

Health maintenance, Alterations in
Related to: Health beliefs

Home maintenance management, Impaired
Related to: Disease of family member other than patient, Home environment obstacles, Inadequate support system, Insufficient family organization or planning

Injury, Potential for
Related to: Sensory deficit

Knowledge deficit
Related to: Limited understanding of disease process, Limited understanding of prescribed treatment

Noncompliance
Related to: Negative consequence of treatment regimen, Negative perception of treatment regimen, Dysfunctional relationship with health care providers

Nutrition, Alteration in: Less than body requirements
Related to: Inadequate nutrition, Nausea and vomiting

Nutrition, Alteration in: More than body requirements
Related to: Ingestion of intake greater than metabolic requirement

Self-concept, Disturbance in
Related to: Body image, Self-esteem, Role performance

Sexual dysfunction
Related to: Altered bladder control, Depression, Impotence, Medications

Skin integrity, Impairment of
Related to: Altered sensation, Draining wound, Long-term steroid therapy

Tissue perfusion, Alteration in
Related to: Impaired circulation

Gastrointestinal bleed

Anxiety
Related to: Specific to patient

Bowel elimination, Alteration in: Diarrhea
Related to: Disease process, Medications, Stress

Comfort, Alteration in:
Related to: Pain

Coping, Ineffective individual
Related to: Anger, Anxiety, Depression

Fear
Related to: Disease process, Hospitalization, Invasive medical procedures, Powerlessness, Real or imagined threat to well-being

Fluid volume deficit
Related to: Abnormal fluid loss, Decreased fluid intake

Health maintenance, Alterations in
Related to: Health beliefs

Home maintenance management, Impaired
Related to: Disease of family member other than patient, Home environment obstacles, Inadequate support system, Insufficient family organization or planning

Knowledge deficit
Related to: Limited understanding of disease treatment, Limited understanding of prescribed treatment

Noncompliance
Related to: Negative consequence of treatment regimen, Dysfunctional relationship with health care providers

Nutrition, Alteration in: Less than body requirements
Related to: Inadequate nutrition, Loss of appetite, Nausea and vomiting

Self-concept, Disturbance in
Related to: Body image, Personal identity, Role performance, Self-esteem

Skin integrity, Impairment of
Related to: Incontinence (stool)

Sleep pattern disturbance
Related to: Sleep deprivation

Immobilized patient

Activity intolerance
Related to: Weakness/fatigue

Anxiety
Related to: Specific to patient

Bowel elimination, Alteration in: Constipation
Related to: Decreased activity, Medications

Comfort, Alteration in
Related to: Pain

Coping, Ineffective individual
Related to: Anger, Anxiety, Depression

Diversional activity deficit
Related to: Boredom

Immobilized patient *(continued)*

Fear
Related to: Disease process, Hospitalization, Powerlessness, Real or imagined threat to well-being

Mobility, Impaired physical
Related to: Decreased strength and endurance, Musculoskeletal impairment

Noncompliance
Related to: Dysfunctional relationship with health care providers

Powerlessness
Related to: Hospitalization

Respiratory functions, Alteration in: Airway clearance, ineffective
Related to: Specific to patient

Self-care deficit
Related to: Inability/limitations in: feeding, bathing/hygiene, dressing/grooming, toileting

Self-concept, Disturbance in
Related to: Body image, Role performance

Sensory-perceptual alterations
Related to: Sensory overload

Skin integrity, Impairment of
Related to: Altered sensation, Pressure ulcer

Sleep pattern disturbance
Related to: Sleep deprivation

Tissue perfusion, Impairment of
Related to: Impaired circulation

Urinary elimination, Alteration in pattern
Related to: Specific to patient

Infection

Activity intolerance
Related to: Weakness and fatigue

Anxiety
Related to: Specific to patient

Bowel elimination, Alteration in: Diarrhea
Related to: Medications

Cardiac output, Alteration in: Decreased
Related to: Stress on heart's function

Comfort, Alteration in
Related to: Pain

Coping, Ineffective individual
Related to: Anxiety, Denial, Depression

Diversional activity deficit
Related to: Boredom

Fear
Related to: Disease process, Hospitalization, Invasive medical procedures, Powerlessness, Real or imagined threat to well-being, Surgical procedure

Fluid volume deficit
Related to: Abnormal fluid loss, Decreased fluid intake

Injury, Potential for
Related to: Specific to patient

Knowledge deficit
Related to: Limited understanding of prescribed treatment

Nutrition, Alteration in: Less than body requirements
Related to: Inadequate nutrition, Nausea and vomiting

Respiratory functions, Alteration in: Breathing pattern, ineffective
Related to: Specific to patient

Skin integrity, Impairment of
Related to: Altered sensation, Draining wound, Immobility, Incontinence (stool, urine), Pressure ulcer, Stomal problems

Sleep pattern disturbance
Related to: Sleep deprivation

Social isolation
Related to: Medical condition

Thought process, Alteration in
Related to: Impaired perception of reality

Urinary elimination, Alteration in pattern
Related to: Specific to patient

Liver disease

Includes, but is not limited to: Cirrhosis; Hepatitis.

Activity intolerance
Related to: Weakness/fatigue

Anxiety
Related to: Specific to patient

Bowel elimination, Alteration in: Constipation
Related to: Decreased activity, Decreased fluid intake, Dietary changes, Medications

Bowel elimination, Alteration in: Diarrhea
Related to: Dietary changes, Medications, Stress

Cardiac output, Alteration in: Decreased
Related to: Arrhythmia, Stress on heart's function, Drug intolerance

Comfort, Alteration in
Related to: Pain

Coping, Ineffective individual
Related to: Anger, Anxiety, Denial, Dependent behavior, Depression

Family process, Alteration in
Related to: Change in family roles, Complex therapies, Illness of family member

Fear
Related to: Disease process, Hospitalization, Invasive medical procedures, Powerlessness, Real or imagined threat to well-being

Fluid volume, Alteration in: Excess
Related to: Ascites

Fluid volume deficit
Related to: Abnormal fluid loss, Decreased fluid intake

Grieving
Related to: Actual or perceived loss

Health maintenance, Alterations in
Related to: Health beliefs

Injury, Potential for
Related to: Substance intoxication, Psychomotor hyperactivity

Knowledge deficit
Related to: Limited understanding of prescribed treatment

Mobility, Impaired physical
Related to: Decreased strength and endurance

Nutrition, Alteration in: Less than body requirements
Related to: Inadequate nutrition, Loss of appetite, Nausea and vomiting

Respiratory functions, Alteration in: Breathing pattern, ineffective
Related to: Specific to patient

Self-care deficit
Related to: Inability/limitations in: feeding, bathing/hygiene, dressing/grooming, toileting

Self-concept, Disturbance
Related to: Body image, Personal identity, Role performance, Self-esteem

Sensory-perceptual alterations
Related to: Altered consciousness, Sensory overload

Liver disease *(continued)*

Skin integrity, Impairment of
Related to: Immobility

Social isolation
*Related to: Chemical dependency,
Medical condition*

Thought process, Alteration in
*Related to: Impaired perception of
reality*

Tissue perfusion, Alteration in
Related to: Impaired circulation

Myocardial infarction

Activity intolerance
Related to: Pain, Weakness/fatigue

Anxiety
Related to: Specific to patient

**Cardiac output, Alteration in:
Decreased**
*Related to: Arrhythmia, Stress on
heart's function*

Comfort, Alteration in
Related to: Pain

Coping, Ineffective individual
*Related to: Anger, Anxiety, Depen-
dent behavior, Depression*

Family process, Alteration in
*Related to: Change in family roles,
Complex therapies, Hospitalization, Ill-
ness of family member*

Fear
*Related to: Disease process, Hos-
pitalization, Invasive medical procedures, Powerlessness, Real or
imagined threat to well-being*

**Home maintenance management,
Impaired**
*Related to: Home environment ob-
stacles, Inadequate support system,
Insufficient family organization or
planning*

Knowledge deficit
*Related to: Limited understanding of
disease process, Limited understanding of prescribed treatment*

Noncompliance
*Related to: Negative consequence of
treatment regimen, Dysfunctional relationship with health care providers*

Powerlessness
Related to: Hospitalization

**Respiratory functions, Alteration in:
Breathing pattern, ineffective; Gas
exchange, impaired**
Related to: Specific to patient

Self-care deficit
*Related to: Inability/limitation in: bath-
ing/hygiene, dressing/grooming,
toileting*

Self-concept, Disturbance in
*Related to: Personal identity, Role
performance, Self-esteem*

Sexual dysfunction
*Related to: Body image, Depression,
Impotence, Medications*

Sleep pattern disturbance
*Related to: Medications, Sleep depri-
vation*

Tissue perfusion, Alteration in
Related to: Impaired circulation

Neurologic disorders

*Includes, but is not limited to: Multi-
ple Sclerosis; Amyotrophic Lateral
Sclerosis; Brain Tumors; Guillain-
Barré Syndrome; Myasthenia Gravis;
Seizure Disorders; Alzheimer's Dis-
ease.*

Anxiety
Related to: Specific to patient

Bowel elimination, Alteration in: Constipation
Related to: Decreased activity, Others specific to patient

Bowel elimination, Alteration in: Incontinence
Related to: Disease process, Decreased awareness of need to defecate, Others specific to patient

Comfort, Alteration in
Related to: Pain (chronic), Others specific to patient

Communication, Impaired: Verbal
Related to: Acute confusion, Inability to speak, Aphasia (expressive and receptive), Others specific to patient

Coping, Ineffective individual
Related to: Anger, Dependent behavior, Depression, Others specific to patient

Family process, Alteration in
Related to: Change in family roles, Complex therapies, Hospitalization, Others specific to patient

Fear
Related to: Disease process, Hospitalization, Real or imagined threat to well-being, Others specific to patient

Home maintenance management, Impaired
Related to: Inadequate support system, Insufficient family organization or planning, Others specific to patient

Injury, Potential for
Related to: Motor deficit, Sensory deficit, Psychomotor hyperactivity, Others specific to patient

Knowledge deficit
Related to: Limited understanding of disease process, Limited understanding of prescribed treatment, Others specific to patient

Mobility, Impaired physical
Related to: Decreased strength and endurance, Musculoskeletal impairment, Neuromuscular impairment, Others specific to patient

Nutrition, Alteration in: Less than body requirements
Related to: Difficulty swallowing, Inadequate nutrition, Others specific to patient

Respiratory functions, Alteration in: Airway clearance, ineffective; Breathing pattern, ineffective; Mechanical ventilation
Related to: Disease process, Others specific to patient

Self-care deficit
Related to: Inability/limitation in; feeding, bathing/hygiene, dressing/grooming, toileting, Others specific to patient

Self-concept, Disturbance in
Related to: Body image, Personal identity, Role performance, Self-esteem, Others specific to patient

Sensory-perceptual alterations
Related to: Altered consciousness, Others specific to patient

Skin integrity, Impairment of
Related to: Immobility, Incontinence (stool, urine), Altered sensation, Others specific to patient

Social isolation
Related to: Medical condition, Others specific to patient

Spiritual distress
Related to: Disruption in spiritual practices, Test of spiritual beliefs, Others specific to patient

Thought process, Alteration in
Related to: Impaired perception of reality, Psychological changes related to aging, Others specific to patient

Neurologic disorders *(continued)*

Urinary elimination, Alteration in pattern
Related to: Specific to patient

Pancreatitis
■────────────────────

Activity intolerance
Related to: Pain, Weakness and fatigue

Anxiety
Related to: Specific to patient

Bowel elimination, Alteration in: Diarrhea
Related to: Disease process, Medications

Comfort, Alteration in
Related to: Pain

Coping, Ineffective individual
Related to: Anger, Anxiety, Depression

Family process, Alteration in
Related to: Complex therapies, Hospitalization, Illness of family member

Fear
Related to: Disease process, Hospitalization, Invasive medical procedures, Powerlessness, Real or imagined threat to well-being

Fluid volume deficit
Related to: Abnormal fluid loss, Decreased fluid intake

Health maintenance, Alterations in
Related to: Health beliefs

Knowledge deficit
Related to: Limited understanding of disease process

Noncompliance
Related to: Dysfunctional relationship with health care providers, Negative perception of treatment regimen

Nutrition, Alteration in: Less than body requirements
Related to: Inadequate nutrition, Loss of appetite, Nausea and vomiting

Respiratory functions, Alteration in: Breathing pattern, ineffective
Related to: Specific to patient

Self-care deficit
Related to: Inability/limitations in: feeding, bathing/hygiene, dressing/grooming, toileting

Self-concept, Disturbance in
Related to: Body image, Personal identity, Role performance, Self-esteem

Sleep pattern disturbance
Related to: Sleep deprivation

Thought process, Alteration in
Related to: Impaired judgment of reality

Pericarditis, endocarditis
■────────────────────

Anxiety
Related to: Specific to patient

Cardiac output, Alteration in: Decreased
Related to: Stress on heart's function

Comfort, Alteration in
Related to: Pain

Coping, Ineffective individual
Related to: Anxiety, Depression

Diversional activity deficit
Related to: Boredom

Fear
Related to: Disease process, Hospitalization, Invasive medical procedures, Powerlessness, Real or imagined threat to well-being

Home maintenance management, Impaired
Related to: Home environment obstacles, Insufficient family organization or planning

Powerlessness
Related to: Hospitalization

Respiratory functions, Alteration in: Breathing pattern, ineffective
Related to: Specific to patient

Pneumonia

Please see Nursing Diagnosis list under medical condition Infection.

Activity intolerance
Related to: Weakness and fatigue

Anxiety
Related to: Specific to patient

Comfort, Alteration in
Related to: Pain

Coping, Ineffective individual
Related to: Anxiety, Dependent behavior

Fear
Related to: Disease process, Hospitalization, Invasive medical procedures, Powerlessness, Real or imagined threat to well-being

Fluid volume deficit
Related to: Abnormal fluid loss, Decreased fluid intake

Knowledge deficit
Related to: Limited understanding of prescribed treatment

Nutrition, Alteration in: Less than body requirements
Related to: Loss of appetite

Respiratory functions, Alteration in: Airway clearance, ineffective; Breathing pattern, ineffective; Gas exchange, impaired
Related to: Specific to patient

Self-care deficit
Related to: Inability/limitations in: feeding, bathing/hygiene, dressing/ grooming, toileting

Skin integrity, Impairment of
Related to: Immobility

Sleep pattern disturbance
Related to: Sleep deprivation

Pulmonary edema

Activity intolerance
Related to: Impaired gas exchange, Weakness and fatigue

Anxiety
Related to: Specific to patient

Cardiac output, Alteration in: Decreased
Related to: Arrhythmias, Stress on heart's function

Coping, Ineffective individual
Related to: Anxiety

Fear
Related to: Disease process, Hospitalization, Invasive medical procedures, Powerlessness, Real or imagined threat to well-being

Fluid volume, Alteration in: Excess
Related to: Specific to patient

Health maintenance, Alterations in
Related to: Health beliefs

Noncompliance
Related to: Negative consequence of treatment regimen

Pulmonary edema *(continued)*

Nutrition, Alteration in: Less than body requirements
Related to: Inadequate nutrition, Loss of appetite

Respiratory functions, Alteration in: Breathing pattern, ineffective; Gas exchange, impaired
Related to: Specific to patient

Self-care deficit
Related to: Inability/limitations in: feeding, bathing/hygiene, dressing/ grooming, toileting

Skin integrity, Impairment of
Related to: Immobility

Sleep pattern disturbance
Related to: Sleep deprivation

Urinary elimination, Alteration in pattern
Related to: Specific to patient

Pulmonary embolism
■────────────────

Activity intolerance
Related to: Impaired gas exchange, Pain, Weakness/fatigue

Anxiety
Related to: Specific to patient

Cardiac output, Alteration in: Decreased
Related to: Arrhythmias, Stress on heart's function

Comfort, Alteration in
Related to: Pain

Coping, Ineffective individual
Related to: Anxiety

Diversional activity deficit
Related to: Boredom

Fear
Related to: Disease process, Hospitalization, Invasive medical procedures, Powerlessness, Real or imagined threat to well-being

Knowledge deficit
Related to: Limited understanding of prescribed treatment

Powerlessness
Related to: Hospitalization

Respiratory functions, Alteration in: Gas exchange, impaired
Related to: Specific to patient

Self-care deficit
Related to: Inability/limitations in: feeding, bathing/hygiene, dressing/ grooming, toileting

Sleep pattern disturbance
Related to: Sleep deprivation

Renal failure, acute
■────────────────

Anxiety
Related to: Specific to patient

Cardiac output, Alteration in: Decreased
Related to: Arrhythmia, Drug intolerance, Stress on the heart's function

Comfort, Alteration in
Related to: Infection, Muscle cramps, Pain (acute)

Coping, Ineffective individual
Related to: Anger, Anxiety, Denial, Dependent behavior, Depression

Family process, Alteration in
Related to: Complex therapies, Hospitalization, Illness of family member

Fear
Related to: Disease process, Hospitalization, Invasive medical procedures, Powerlessness, Real or imagined threat to well-being

Fluid volume, Alteration in: Excess
Related to: Increased intake, Decreased output

Fluid volume deficit
Related to: Abnormal fluid loss, Decreased fluid intake

Grieving
Related to: Actual or perceived loss, Anticipated loss

Knowledge deficit
Related to: Limited understanding of disease process, Limited understanding of prescribed treatment

Nutrition, Alteration in: Less than body requirements
Related to: Dietary restrictions, Loss of appetite, Nausea and vomiting

Powerlessness
Related to: Disease process, Hospitalization

Respiratory functions, Alteration in: Breathing pattern, ineffective; Gas exchange, impaired
Related to: Fluid overload

Self-concept, Disturbance in
Related to: Body image, Personal identity, Role performance, Self-esteem

Thought process, Alteration in
Related to: Impaired perception of reality

Urinary elimination, Alteration in pattern
Related to: Decreased kidney function, Decreased urine output

Renal failure, chronic

Activity intolerance
Related to: Weakness and fatigue

Anxiety
Related to: Specific to patient

Bowel elimination, Alteration in: Constipation
Related to: Medication

Cardiac output, Alteration in: Decreased
Related to: Arrhythmia, Drug intolerance, Stress on the heart's function

Comfort, Alteration in
Related to: Infection, Muscle cramps, Pain (chronic)

Communication, Impaired: Verbal
Related to: Acute confusion, Primary language other than English

Coping, Ineffective individual
Related to: Anger, Anxiety, Denial, Dependent behavior, Depression

Diversional activity deficit
Related to: Boredom

Family process, Alteration in
Related to: Complex therapies, Illness of family member

Fear
Related to: Disease process, Hospitalization, Invasive medical procedures, Powerlessness, Real or imagined threat to well-being

Fluid volume, Alteration in: Excess
Related to: Increased intake, Decreased output

Fluid volume deficit
Related to: Abnormal fluid loss, Decreased fluid intake

Grieving
Related to: Actual loss of kidney function, Perceived loss of control, independence

Health maintenance, Alterations in
Related to: Health beliefs

Renal failure *(continued)*

Home maintenance management, Impaired
Related to: Disease of family member, Home situation obstacles, Inadequate support system, Insufficient family organization or planning

Injury, Potential for
Related to: Hypotension, Motor deficit, Sensory deficit

Knowledge deficit
Related to: Limited understand of prescribed treatment

Mobility, Impaired physical
Related to: Decreased strength and endurance, Musculoskeletal impairment, Neuromuscular impairment

Noncompliance
Related to: Dysfunctional relationship with health care providers, Negative consequence of treatment regimen, Negative perception of treatment regimen

Nutrition, Alteration in: Less than body requirements
Related to: Loss of appetite, Nausea and vomiting

Powerlessness
Related to: Disease process, Hospitalization

Respiratory functions, Alteration in: Breathing pattern, ineffective; Gas exchange, impaired
Related to: Anemia, Volume overload

Self-care deficit
Related to: Inability/limitations in: feeding, bathing/hygiene, dressing/grooming, toileting

Self-concept, Disturbance in
Related to: Body image, Personal identity, Role performance, Self-esteem

Sensory-perceptual alterations
Related to: Altered consciousness, Partial/total loss of hearing, Partial/total loss of vision, Physiologic changes related to aging, Sensory overload

Sexual dysfunction
Related to: Body image, Depression, Impotence, Physiological limitations

Skin integrity, Impairment of
Related to: Skin abrasions

Sleep pattern disturbance
Related to: Sleep deprivation

Social isolation
Related to: Chronologic age, Medical condition, Physical handicaps

Spiritual distress
Related to: Disruption in spiritual practices

Thought process, Alteration in
Related to: Impaired perception of reality

Tissue perfusion, Alteration in
Related to: Impaired circulation

Urinary elimination, Alteration in pattern
Related to: Decreased kidney function, Decreased urine output

Substance abuse

Includes, but is not limited to: Drug Abuse; Alcohol Abuse.

Activity intolerance
Related to: Weakness and fatigue

Anxiety
Related to: Specific to patient

Communication, Impaired: Verbal
Related to: Inability to speak

Coping, Ineffective individual
Related to: Aggression, Anger, Anxiety, Denial, Dependent behavior, Depression

Family process, Alteration in
Related to: Change in family roles, Hospitalization

Fear
Related to: Hospitalization, Power-lessness, Real or imagined threat to well-being

Fluid volume, Alteration in: Excess
Related to: Specific to patient

Fluid volume deficit
Related to: Abnormal fluid loss, Decreased fluid intake

Health maintenance, Alterations in
Related to: Health beliefs

Home maintenance management, Impaired
Related to: Home environment obstacles, Insufficient family organization or planning

Injury, Potential for
Related to: Substance intoxication, Psychomotor hyperactivity

Knowledge deficit
Related to: Limited understanding of disease process, Limited understanding of prescribed treatment

Nutrition, Alteration in: Less than body requirements
Related to: Inadequate nutrition, Loss of appetite, Nausea and vomiting

Powerlessness
Related to: Disease process, Hospitalization

Respiratory functions, Alteration in: Breathing pattern, ineffective
Related to: Specific to patient

Sexual dysfunction
Related to: Body image disturbance, Depression, Impotence, Physiological limitations

Self-care deficit
Related to: Inability/limitations in: feeding, bathing/hygiene, dressing/grooming, toileting

Self-concept, Disturbance in
Related to: Body image, Personal identity, Role performance, Self-esteem

Sleep pattern disturbance
Related to: Sleep deprivation

Thought process, Alteration in
Related to: Impaired judgment of reality

Violence, Potential for
Related to: Impaired behavior patterns

Terminal patient

■

Activity intolerance
Related to: Pain, Weakness/fatigue

Anxiety
Related to: Specific to patient

Bowel elimination, Alteration in: Constipation
Related to: Decreased activity, Medications

Bowel elimination, Alteration in: Diarrhea
Related to: Disease process

Bowel elimination, Alteration in: Incontinence
Related to: Disease process

Comfort, Alteration in
Related to: Pain

Communication, Impaired: Verbal
Related to: Inability to speak

Terminal patient *(continued)*

Coping, Ineffective individual
Related to: Anger, Anxiety, Denial, Dependent behavior, Depression

Family process, Alteration in
Related to: Care of elderly family member, Change in family roles, Hospitalization, Illness of family member

Fear
Related to: Disease process, Dying, Hospitalization, Powerlessness, Real or imagined threat to well-being

Fluid volume, Alteration in: Excess
Related to: Specific to patient

Fluid volume deficit
Related to: Decreased fluid intake

Grieving
Related to: Actual or perceived loss, Anticipated loss

Health maintenance, Alterations in: Impaired
Related to: Health beliefs

Home maintenance management, Impaired
Related to: Disease of family member other than patient, Home environment obstacles, Inadequate support system, Insufficient family organization or planning

Mobility, Impaired physical
Related to: Decreased strength and endurance, Musculoskeletal impairment

Nutrition, Alteration in: Less than body requirements
Related to: Difficulty swallowing, Inadequate nutrition, Loss of appetite, Nausea and vomiting

Oral mucous membranes, Alteration in
Related to: Insufficient oral hygiene, Stomatitis

Powerlessness
Related to: Dying process, Hospitalization

Respiratory functions, Alteration in: Airway clearance, ineffective; Breathing pattern, ineffective; Gas exchange, impaired
Related to: Specific to patient

Self-care deficit
Related to: Inability/limitations in: feeding, bathing/hygiene, dressing/grooming, toileting

Self-concept, Disturbance in
Related to: Body image, Personal identity, Role performance, Self-esteem

Sensory-perceptual alterations
Related to: Altered consciousness, Physiologic changes related to aging, Sensory overload, Terminal illness

Skin integrity, Impairment of
Related to: Draining wound, Immobility, Incontinence (stool, urine), Pressure ulcer

Sleep pattern disturbance
Related to: Sleep deprivation

Social isolation
Related to: Medical condition

Spiritual distress
Related to: Discrepancy between spiritual beliefs and prescribed treatment, Disruption in spiritual practices, Test of spiritual beliefs

Thought process, Alteration in
Related to: Impaired perception of reality

Tissue perfusion, Alteration in
Related to: Impaired circulation

Urinary elimination, Alteration in pattern
Related to: Specific to patient

Urologic disorders
∎━━━━━━━━━━━━━━━━━━━━━

Includes, but is not limited to: Cystitis; Glomerulonephritis; Pyelonephritis; Urolithiasis.

Anxiety
Related to: Specific to patient

Comfort, Alteration in
Related to: Pain (acute), Others specific to patient

Fear
Related to: Disease process, Invasive medical procedure, Others specific to patient

Knowledge deficit
Related to: Limited understanding of disease process, Limited understanding of prescribed treatment, Others specific to patient

Urinary elimination, Alteration in
Related to: Specific to patient

Vascular disease
∎━━━━━━━━━━━━━━━━━━━━━

Includes, but is not limited to: Deep Vein Thrombosis; Hypertension; Stasis Ulcers; Varicosities.

Activity intolerance
Related to: Weakness and fatigue, Pain, Others specific to patient

Anxiety
Related to: Specific to patient

Comfort, Alteration in
Related to: Pain (acute), Others specific to patient

Fear
Related to: Disease process, Others specific to patient

Health maintenance, Alterations in
Related to: Specific to patient

Injury, Potential for
Related to: Sensory deficit, Hypotension, Others specific to patient

Knowledge deficit
Related to: Limited understanding of disease process, Limited understanding of prescribed treatment

Noncompliance
Related to: Negative perception of treatment regimen, Others specific to patient

Self-care deficit
Related to: Inability/limitation in: bathing/hygiene, toileting, Others specific to patient

Self-concept, Disturbance in
Related to: Body image, Others specific to patient

Skin integrity, Impairment of
Related to: Pressure ulcer, Draining wound, Altered sensation, Immobility, Others specific to patient

Tissue perfusion, Alteration in
Related to: Impaired circulation, Others specific to patient

Surgical Conditions

Abdominal surgery

Includes, but is not limited to: Appendectomy; Cholecystectomy; Colectomy; Colon Resection; Colostomy; Gastrectomy; Gastric Resection, Gastroenterostomy; Hysterectomy; Ileostomy; Laparotomy; Lysis of Adhesions; Marshall-Marchetti Procedure; Ovarian Cystectomy; Salpingotomy; Small Bowel Resection; Splenectomy; Vagotomy.

Anxiety
Related to: Specific to patient

Bowel elimination, Alteration in: Constipation
Related to: Decreased activity, Dietary changes, Medications, Painful defecation

Bowel elimination, Alteration in: Diarrhea
Related to: Dietary changes, Disease process, Impaction, Medication, Stress

Bowel elimination, Alteration in: Incontinence
Related to: Disease process, Loss of sphincter control

Comfort, Alteration in
Related to: Pain

Coping, Ineffective individual
Related to: Anxiety, Depression

Fear
Related to: Disease process, Hospitalization, Powerlessness, Real or imagined threat to well-being, Surgical procedure

Fluid volume deficit
Related to: Abnormal fluid loss, Decreased fluid intake

Knowledge deficit
Related to: Limited understanding of prescribed treatment

Mobility impaired, Physical
Related to: Decreased strength and endurance

Nutrition, Alteration in: Less than body requirements
Related to: Inadequate nutrition, Loss of appetite, Nausea and vomiting

Respiratory functions, Alteration in: Airway clearance, ineffective; Breathing pattern, ineffective; Gas exchange, impaired
Related to: Specific to patient

Self-concept, Disturbance in
Related to: Body image, Personal identity

Sexual dysfunction
Related to: Depression, Physiologic limitations

Skin integrity, Impairment of
Related to: Draining wound, Stomal problems

Breast surgery

Includes, but is not limited to: Augmentation; Biopsy; Lumpectomy; Mastectomy; Reconstruction.

Activity intolerance
Related to: Pain, Weakness/fatigue

Anxiety
Related to: Specific to patient

Comfort, Alteration in
Related to: Pain

Coping, Ineffective individual
Related to: Anger, Anxiety, Denial, Dependent behavior, Depression

Family process, Alteration in
Related to: Complex therapies, Hospitalization

Fear
Related to: Disease process, Hospitalization, Powerlessness, Real or imagined threat to well-being, Surgical procedure

Fluid volume deficit
Related to: Abnormal fluid loss, Decreased fluid intake

Grieving
Related to: Actual loss, Anticipated loss, Perceived loss

Home maintenance management, Impaired
Related to: Home environment obstacles, Inadequate support system

Knowledge deficit
Related to: Limited understanding of disease process, Limited understanding of prescribed treatment

Nutrition, Alteration in: Less than body requirements
Related to: Loss of appetite, Nausea and vomiting

Self-care deficit
Related to: Inability/limitation in: bathing/hygiene, dressing/grooming

Self-concept, Disturbance in
Related to: Body image, Personal identity, Role performance, Self-esteem

Sexual dysfunction
Related to: Body image, Depression, Physiologic limitations

Sleep pattern disturbance
Related to: Sleep deprivation

Spiritual distress
Related to: Test of spiritual beliefs

Chest surgery

Includes, but is not limited to: Biopsy; Cardiopulmonary Bypass; Coronary Artery Bypass; Lobectomy; Thoracotomy.

Activity intolerance
Related to: Pain, Weakness and fatigue

Anxiety
Related to: Specific to patient

Cardiac output, Alteration in: Decreased
Related to: Drug side-effects, Stress on heart's function

Comfort, Alteration in
Related to: Pain

Coping, Ineffective individual
Related to: Anxiety

Fear
Related to: Disease process, Hospitalization, Powerlessness, Real or imagined threat to well-being, Surgical procedure

Fluid volume deficit
Related to: Abnormal fluid loss, Decreased fluid intake

Knowledge deficit
Related to: Limited understanding of disease process, Limited understanding of prescribed treatment

Mobility, Impaired physical
Related to: Decreased strength and endurance

Powerlessness
Related to: Hospitalization

Respiratory functions, Alteration in: Airway clearance, ineffective; Breathing pattern, ineffective; Gas exchange, impaired
Related to: Specific to patient

Chest surgery *(continued)*

Self-care activities
Related to: Inability/limitation in: feeding, bathing/hygiene, dressing/ grooming, toileting

Self-concept, Disturbance in
Related to: Body image, Role performance

Sleep pattern disturbance
Related to: Sleep deprivation

Tissue perfusion, Alteration in
Related to: Impaired circulation

Craniotomy

Includes, but is not limited to: Acoustic Neuroma Removal; Cerebral Aneurysm Clipping.

Anxiety
Related to: Specific to patient

Comfort, Alteration in
Related to: Pain

Communication, Impaired: Verbal
Related to: Inability to speak

Coping, Ineffective individual
Related to: Anger, Anxiety, Denial, Dependent behavior, Depression

Family process, Alteration in
Related to: Complex therapies, Hospitalization, Illness of family member

Fear
Related to: Disease process, Hospitalization, Powerlessness, Real or imagined threat to well-being, Surgical procedure

Fluid volume, Alteration in: Excess
Related to: Specific to patient

Home maintenance management, Impaired
Related to: Home environment obstacles, Inadequate support system, Insufficient family organization or planning

Injury, Potential for
Related to: Hypotension, Motor deficit, Sensory deficit

Knowledge deficit
Related to: Limited understanding of prescribed treatment

Mobility, Impaired physical
Related to: Decreased strength and endurance, Neuromuscular impairment

Nutrition, Alteration in: Less than body requirements
Related to: Loss of appetite, Nausea and vomiting

Self-care deficit
Related to: Inability/limitation in: feeding, bathing/hygiene, dressing/ grooming, toileting

Self-concept, Disturbance in
Related to: Body image, Personal identity, Role performance, Self-esteem

Sensory-perceptual alterations
Related to: Altered consciousness, Sensory overload

Sleep pattern disturbance
Related to: Sleep deprivation

Thought process, Alteration in
Related to: Impaired perception of reality

Urinary elimination, Alteration in pattern
Related to: Specific to patient

Violence, Potential for
Related to: Impaired behavior pattern

Ear surgery
■————————————

Includes, but is not limited to: Myringotomy; Reconstruction; Stapedectomy.

Anxiety
Related to: Specific to patient

Comfort, Alteration in
Related to: Pain

Coping, Ineffective individual
Related to: Anxiety

Fear
Related to: Hospitalization, Powerlessness, Surgical procedure

Injury, Potential for
Related to: Sensory deficit

Knowledge deficit
Related to: Limited understanding of prescribed treatment

Nutrition, Alteration in: Less than body requirements
Related to: Nausea and vomiting

Self-concept, Disturbance in
Related to: Body image

Sensory-perceptual alterations
Related to: Partial/total loss of hearing, Sensory overload

Sleep pattern disturbance
Related to: Sleep deprivation

Eye surgery
■————————————

Includes, but is not limited to: Blepharoplasty; Cataract Removal; Cryosurgery for Retinal Detachment; Iridectomy; Iridotomy; Lens Implant.

Anxiety
Related to: Specific to patient

Comfort, Alteration in
Related to: Pain

Coping, Ineffective individual
Related to: Anxiety

Fear
Related to: Hospitalization, Powerlessness, Real or imagined threat to well-being, Surgical procedure

Home maintenance management, Impaired
Related to: Home environment obstacles, Insufficient family organization or planning

Injury, Potential for
Related to: Visual disturbances

Knowledge deficit
Related to: Limited understanding of prescribed treatment

Nutrition, Alteration in: Less than body requirements
Related to: Nausea and vomiting

Sensory-perceptual alterations
Related to: Partial/total loss of vision, Physiologic changes related to aging, Sensory overload

Self-care deficit
Related to: Inability/limitations in: feeding, bathing/hygiene, dressing/grooming, toileting

Sleep pattern disturbance
Related to: Sleep deprivation

Musculoskeletal surgery
■————————————

Includes, but is not limited to: Amputation; Arthrotomy; Bunionectomy; Carpal Tunnel Repair; Hip Pinning; Hip Prosthesis; Open Reduction/Internal Fixation of Fracture; Shoulder Repair; Total Ankle Replacement; Total Hip Replacement; Total Knee Replacement.

Activity intolerance
Related to: Pain

Musculoskeletal surgery *(continued)*

Anxiety
Related to: Specific to patient

Bowel elimination, Alteration in: Constipation
Related to: Decreased activity, Dietary changes, Medications

Comfort, Alteration in
Related to: Bed rest, Pain

Coping, Ineffective individual
Related to: Anger, Anxiety, Depression

Fear
Related to: Disease process, Hospitalization, Powerlessness, Real or imagined threat to well-being, Surgical procedure

Fluid volume deficit
Related to: Abnormal fluid loss

Health maintenance, Alterations in
Related to: Health beliefs

Home maintenance management, Impaired
Related to: Home environment obstacles, Inadequate support system, Insufficient family organization or planning

Injury, Potential for
Related to: Motor deficit

Knowledge deficit
Related to: Limited understanding of prescribed treatment

Mobility, Impaired physical
Related to: Decreased strength and endurance, Musculoskeletal impairment, Neuromuscular impairment

Noncompliance
Related to: Dysfunctional relationship with health care providers, Negative consequence of treatment regimen

Self-care deficit
Related to: Inability/limitations in: feeding, bathing/hygiene, dressing/grooming, toileting

Self-concept, Disturbance in
Related to: Body image, Personal identity, Role performance, Self-esteem

Skin integrity, Impairment of
Related to: Altered sensation, Cast, Edema, Immobility

Sleep pattern disturbance
Related to: Sleep deprivation

Tissue perfusion, Alteration in
Related to: Impaired circulation

Nasal surgery

Includes, but is not limited to: Nasal Septoplasty; Reconstruction; Rhinoplasty; Tumor Excision.

Anxiety
Related to: Specific to patient

Comfort, Alteration in
Related to: Pain

Coping, Ineffective individual
Related to: Anxiety

Fear
Related to: Disease process, Hospitalization, Invasive medical procedure, Powerlessness, Real or imagined threat to well-being, Surgical procedure

Fluid volume deficit
Related to: Abnormal fluid loss

Knowledge deficit
Related to: Limited understanding of prescribed treatment

Nutrition, Alteration in: Less than body requirements
Related to: Nausea and vomiting

**Oral mucous membranes,
Alteration in**
Related to: Insufficient oral hygiene

**Respiratory functions, Alteration in:
Breathing pattern, ineffective**
Related to: Specific to patient

Self-concept, Alteration in
Related to: Body image

Sleep pattern disturbance
Related to: Sleep deprivation

Neck surgery

*Includes, but is not limited to: Carotid
Endarterectomy; Laryngectomy;
Parathyroidectomy; Radical Neck
Dissection; Thyroidectomy; Tonsillec-
tomy; Tracheostomy.*

Anxiety
Related to: Specific to patient

Comfort, Alteration in
Related to: Pain

Communication, Impaired: Verbal
Related to: Inability to speak

Coping, Ineffective individual
Related to: Anxiety

Fear
*Related to: Disease process, Hos-
pitalization, Invasive medical procedures, Powerlessness, Real or
imagined threat to well-being, Surgical
procedure*

Grieving
*Related to: Actual or perceived loss,
Anticipated loss*

**Home maintenance management,
Impaired**
*Related to: Home environment ob-
stacles, Inadequate support system,
Insufficient family organization or
planning*

Knowledge deficit
*Related to: Limited understanding of
prescribed treatment*

**Nutrition, Alteration in: Less than
body requirements**
*Related to: Difficulty swallowing, Loss
of appetite, Nausea and vomiting*

**Oral mucous membranes,
Alteration in**
Related to: Insufficient oral hygiene

**Respiratory functions, Alteration in:
Airway clearance, ineffective**
Related to: Specific to patient

Self-concept, Disturbance in
*Related to: Body image, Personal
identity, Role performance*

Sleep pattern disturbance
Related to: Sleep deprivation

Rectal surgery

*Includes, but is not limited to:
Fissurectomy; Hemorrhoidectomy;
Pilonidal Cystectomy; Polypectomy.*

Anxiety
Related to: Specific to patient

**Bowel elimination, Alteration in:
Constipation**
*Related to: Decreased activity,
Dietary changes, Medications, Painful
defecation*

Comfort, Alteration in
Related to: Pain

Coping, Ineffective individual
Related to: Anxiety

Fear
*Related to: Disease process, Hos-
pitalization, Invasive medical procedures, Powerlessness, Real or
imagined threat to well-being, Surgical
procedure*

Rectal surgery *(continued)*

Knowledge deficit
Related to: Limited understanding of prescribed treatment

Sleep pattern disturbance
Related to: Sleep deprivation

Urinary elimination, Alteration in pattern
Related to: Specific to patient

Skin graft
■

Includes, but is not limited to: Excision of Lesion with Flap; Excision of Lesion with Full Thickness Graft; Excision of Lesion with Split-Thickness Graft; Excision of Lesion with Synthetic Graft.

Activity intolerance
Related to: Pain, Weakness and fatigue

Anxiety
Related to: Specific to patient

Bowel elimination, Alteration in: Constipation
Related to: Decreased activity, Dietary changes, Medications

Comfort, Alteration in
Related to: Bed rest, Pain

Coping, Ineffective individual
Related to: Anger, Anxiety, Dependent behavior

Fear
Related to: Disease process, Hospitalization, Invasive medical procedures, Powerlessness, Real or imagined threat to well-being, Surgical procedure

Fluid volume deficit
Related to: Abnormal fluid loss

Home maintenance management, Impaired
Related to: Inadequate support system, Insufficient family organization or planning

Knowledge deficit
Related to: Limited understanding of prescribed treatment

Nutrition, Alteration in: Less than body requirements
Related to: Loss of appetite, Nausea and vomiting

Powerlessness
Related to: Hospitalization

Self-care deficit
Related to: Inability/limitations in: feeding, bathing/hygiene, dressing/grooming, toileting

Self-concept, Disturbance in
Related to: Body image, Role performance

Sleep pattern disturbance
Related to: Sleep deprivation

Skin integrity, Impairment of
Related to: Draining wound

Tissue perfusion, Alteration in
Related to: Impaired circulation

Spinal surgery
■

Includes, but is not limited to: Harrington Rod Implant; Laminectomy; Low Back Pain; Luque Rod Implant; Spinal Fusion.

Activity intolerance
Related to: Anxiety, Weakness/fatigue

Anxiety
Related to: Specific to patient

Bowel elimination, Alteration in: Constipation
Related to: Decreased activity, Dietary changes, Medications

Comfort, Alteration in
Related to: Bed rest, Pain

Coping, Ineffective individual
Related to: Anxiety, Depression

Family process, Alteration in
Related to: Complex therapies, Hospitalization

Fear
Related to: Disease process, Hospitalization, Powerlessness, Real or imagined threat to well-being, Surgical procedure

Home maintenance management, Impaired
Related to: Insufficient family organization or planning

Knowledge deficit
Related to: Limited understanding of prescribed treatment

Mobility, Impaired physical
Related to: Decreased strength and endurance, Musculoskeletal impairment, Neuromuscular impairment

Noncompliance
Related to: Dysfunctional relationship with health care provider, Negative consequence of treatment regimen, Negative perception of treatment regimen

Self-care deficit
Related to: Inability/limitations in: feeding, bathing/hygiene, dressing/grooming, toileting

Self-concept, Disturbance in
Related to: Role performance

Skin integrity, Impairment of
Related to: Altered sensation

Sleep pattern disturbance
Related to: Sleep deprivation

Urinary elimination, Alteration in pattern
Related to: Specific to patient

Urologic surgery

Includes, but is not limited to: Anterior/Posterior Repair; Cystoscopy; Nephrectomy; Penile Implant; Percutaneous Nephrostomy; Retroperitoneal Lymphadenotomy; Trans. Urethral Resection of Prostate; Ureterolithotomy; Urostomy; Vasectomy.

Activity intolerance
Related to: Anxiety, Pain, Weakness/fatigue

Anxiety
Related to: Specific to patient

Bowel elimination, Alteration in: Constipation
Related to: Decreased activity, Painful defecation

Comfort, Alteration in
Related to: Pain

Coping, Ineffective individual
Related to: Anxiety, Depression

Fear
Related to: Disease process, Hospitalization, Powerlessness, Real or imagined threat to well-being, Surgical procedure

Fluid volume deficit
Related to: Abnormal fluid loss, Decreased fluid intake

Home maintenance management, Impaired
Related to: Home environment obstacles, Inadequate support system

Knowledge deficit
Related to: Limited understanding of disease process, Limited understanding of prescribed treatment

Urologic surgery *(continued)*

Mobility, Impaired physical
Related to: Musculoskeletal impairment

Self-concept, Disturbance in
Related to: Body image, Role performance, Self-esteem

Sexual dysfunction
Related to: Altered bladder control, Body image, Depression, Impotence, Physiological limitations

Urinary elimination, Alteration in pattern
Related to: Specific to patient

Vascular surgery

■━━━━━━━━━━━━━━━━━━━━━━

Includes, but is not limited to: Aortic Aneurysm Resection; Aorto-iliac Bypass Graft; Embolectomy; Femoral-iliac Bypass Graft; Portacaval Shunt; Sympathectomy; Vein Ligation.

Activity intolerance
Related to: Pain, Weakness/fatigue

Anxiety
Related to: Specific to patient

Bowel elimination, Alteration in: Constipation
Related to: Decreased activity, Medications

Comfort, Alteration in
Related to: Pain

Coping, Ineffective individual
Related to: Anxiety, Denial, Dependent behavior, Depression

Fear
Related to: Disease process, Hospitalization, Invasive medical procedures, Powerlessness, Real or imagined threat to well-being, Surgical procedure

Fluid volume, Alteration in: Excess
Related to: Specific to patient

Knowledge deficit
Related to: Limited understanding of prescribed treatment

Mobility, Impaired physical
Related to: Decreased strength and endurance

Respiratory functions, Alteration in: Breathing pattern, ineffective; Gas exchange, impaired
Related to: Disease process

Self-care deficit
Related to: Inability/limitations in: bathing/hygiene, dressing/grooming, toileting

Self-concept, Disturbance in
Related to: Body image, Role performance

Tissue perfusion, Alteration in
Related to: Impaired circulation

Nursing Diagnoses List

Activity intolerance
Related to: Anxiety, Arrhythmias, Impaired gas exchange, Pain, Weakness/fatigue, Others specific to patient

Anxiety
Related to: Specific to patient

Bowel elimination, Alteration in: Constipation
Related to: Aging process, Decreased activity, Decreased fluid intake, Dietary changes, Disease process, Medications, Painful defecation, Others specific to patient

Bowel elimination, Alteration in: Diarrhea
Related to: Dietary changes, Disease process, Impaction, Medication, Stress, Others specific to patient

Bowel elimination, Alteration in: Incontinence
Related to: Decreased awareness of need to defecate, Disease process, Loss of sphincter control, Others specific to patient

Cardiac output, Alteration in: Decreased
Related to: Arrhythmia, Drug intolerance, Drug side-effects, Stress on heart's function, Others specific to patient

Comfort, Alteration in
Related to: Bed rest, Pain (acute), Pain (chronic), Others specific to patient

Communication, Impaired: Verbal
Related to: Acute confusion, Aphasia (expressive and receptive), Inability to speak, Primary language other than English, Others specific to patient

Coping, Ineffective individual
Related to: Aggression, Anger, Anxiety, Denial, Dependent behavior, Depression, Others specific to patient

Diversional activity deficit
Related to: Boredom, Others specific to patient

Family process, Alteration in
Related to: Care of elderly family member, Change in family roles, Complex therapies, Hospitalization, Illness of family member, Others specific to patient

Fear
Related to: Disease process, Hospitalization, Invasive medical procedures, Real or imagined threat to well-being, Surgical procedure, Others specific to patient

Fluid volume, Alteration in: Excess
Related to: Specific to patient

Fluid volume deficit
Related to: Abnormal fluid loss, Decreased fluid intake, Others specific to patient

Grieving
Related to: Actual or perceived loss, Anticipated loss, Others specific to patient

Health maintenance, Alterations in
Related to: Health beliefs, Others specific to patient

Home maintenance management, Impaired
Related to: Disease of family member other than patient, Home environment obstacles, Inadequate support system, Insufficient family organization or planning, Others specific to patient

Injury, Potential for
Related to: Hypotension, Motor deficit, Psychomotor hyperactivity, Sensory deficit, Substance intoxication, Others specific to patient

Knowledge deficit
Related to: Limited understanding of disease process, Limited understanding of prescribed treatment, Others specific to patient.

Mobility, Impaired physical
Related to: Decreased strength and endurance, Musculoskeletal impairment, Neuromuscular impairment, Others specific to patient

Noncompliance
Related to: Dysfunctional relationship with health care providers, Negative consequence of treatment regimen, Negative perception of treatment regimen, Others specific to patient

Nutrition, Alteration in: Less than body requirements
Related to: Difficulty swallowing, High metabolic states, Inadequate nutrition, Loss of appetite, Nausea and vomiting, Others specific to patient

Nutrition, Alteration in: More than body requirements
Related to: Intake greater than metabolic requirement, Others specific to patient

Oral mucous membranes, Alteration in
Related to: Insufficient oral hygiene, Stomatitis, Others specific to patient

Powerlessness
Related to: Disease process, Hospitalization, Others specific to patient

Respiratory functions, Alteration in: Airway clearance, ineffective; Breathing pattern, ineffective; Gas exchange, impaired; Mechanical ventilation
Related to: Disease process, Others specific to patient

Self-care deficit
Related to: Inability/limitation in: feeding, bathing/hygiene, dressing/ grooming, toileting, Others specific to patient

Self-concept, Disturbance in
Related to: Body image, Personal identity, Role performance, Self-esteem, Others specific to patient

Sensory-perceptual alterations
Related to: Altered consciousness, Partial/total loss of hearing, Partial/ total loss of vision, Physiologic changes related to aging, Sensory overload, Others specific to patient

Sexual dysfunction
Related to: Altered bladder control, Body image disturbance, Depression, Impotence, Medications, Physiologic limitations, Others specific to patient

Skin integrity, Impairment of
Related to: Altered sensation, Draining wound, Immobility, Incontinence (stool, urine), Long-term steroid therapy, Pressure ulcer, Stomal problems, Others specific to patient

Sleep pattern disturbance
Related to: Medication use, Sleep deprivation, Others specific to patient

Social isolation
Related to: Chemical dependency, Chronologic age, Medical condition, Physical handicaps, Sexual preference, Others specific to patient

Spiritual distress
Related to: Discrepancy between spiritual beliefs and prescribed treatment, Disruption in spiritual practices, Test of spiritual beliefs, Others specific to patient

Thought process, Alteration in
Related to: Impaired perception of reality, Psychological changes related to aging, Others specific to patient

Tissue perfusion, Alteration in
Related to: Impaired circulation, Others specific to patient

Urinary elimination, Alteration in pattern
Related to: Specific to patient

Violence, Potential for
Related to: Impaired behavior patterns, Others specific to patient

Approved Nursing Diagnoses

■

North American Nursing Diagnosis Association (NANDA)

Activity intolerance
Activity intolerance, Potential
* Airway clearance, Ineffective
Anxiety
Bowel elimination, Alteration in: Constipation
Bowel elimination, Alteration in: Diarrhea
Bowel elimination, Alteration in: Incontinence
* Breathing pattern, Ineffective
Cardiac output, Alteration in: Decreased
Comfort, Alteration in: Pain
Communication, Impaired: Verbal
Coping, Family: Potential for growth
Coping, Ineffective family: Compromised
Coping, Ineffective family: Disabling
Coping, Ineffective individual
Diversional activity deficit
Family process, Alteration in
Fear
Fluid volume, Alteration in: Excess
Fluid volume deficit, Actual
Fluid volume deficit, Potential
* Gas exchange, Impaired
Grieving, Anticipatory
Grieving, Dysfunctional
Health maintenance, Alterations in
Home maintenance management, Impaired
Injury, Potential for
Knowledge deficit
Mobility, Impaired physical
Noncompliance
Nutrition, Alteration in: Less than body requirements
Nutrition, Alteration in: More than body requirements

Indicates respiratory diagnosis by NANDA

Approved nursing diagnoses (continued)

Nutrition, Alteration in, Potential for more than body requirement

Oral mucous membranes, Alteration in

Parenting, Alteration in: Actual

Parenting, Alteration in: Potential

Powerlessness

Rape trauma syndrome

*Respiratory functions, Alteration in: Airway clearance, ineffective; Breathing pattern, ineffective; Gas exchange, impaired; Mechanical ventilation

Self-care deficit: Feeding, bathing/hygiene, dressing/grooming, toileting

Self-concept, Disturbance in: Body image, self-esteem, role performance, personal identity

Sensory-perceptual alterations: Visual, auditory, kinesthetic, gustatory, tactile, olfactory

Sexual dysfunction

Skin integrity, Impairment of: Actual

Skin integrity, Impairment of: Potential

Sleep pattern disturbance

Social isolation

Spiritual distress

Thought process, Alteration in

Tissue perfusion, Alteration in: Cerebral, cardiopulmonary, renal, gastrointestinal, peripheral

Urinary elimination, Alteration in pattern

Violence, Potential for: Self-directed or directed at others

■————————————————————————————————

Indicates composite diagnosis of Respiratory Function; alterations added for ECH publication by Publishing Task Force.

Bibliography

Bockrath M: Your patient needs two diagnoses: Medical and nursing. *Nursing Life* March/April 1982; 2: 29–32.

Carlson J, Craft C, McGuire A: *Nursing diagnosis.* Philadelphia: Saunders, 1982.

Carpenito LJ: *Nursing diagnosis: Applications to clinical practice.* Philadelphia: Lippincott, 1983.

Carpenito LJ: Diagnostics: Is the problem a nursing diagnosis? *American Journal of Nursing* 1984; 84: 11.

Carpenito LJ: *Handbook of nursing diagnoses.* Philadelphia: Lippincott, 1984.

Gebbie K: Nursing diagnosis: What is it and why does it exist? *Topics in Clinical Nursing* January 1984; 5(4): 1–9.

Gettrust K, Ryan S, and Engelman D: *Applied nursing diagnosis: Guides for comprehensive care planning.* New York: Wiley, 1985.

Gordon, MJ: *Manual of nursing diagnoses.* New York: McGraw-Hill, 1985.

Gordon M, Sweeney M, McKeehan K: Nursing diagnosis: Looking at its use in the clinical area. *American Journal of Nursing* 1980; 80: 672–74.

Jones P, Jakob D: Nursing diagnosis: Differentiating fear and anxiety. *Nursing Papers* 1981; 13: 20.

Kieffer J: Nursing diagnosis can make a critical difference. *Nursing Life* May/June 1984; 4(3): 18–21.

Kim MJ, McFarland GK, McLane AM (editors): *Classification of nursing diagnoses: Proceedings of the Fifth National Conference.* Saint Louis: Mosby, 1984.

Kim MJ, McFarland GK, McLane AM: *Pocket guide to nursing diagnoses.* Saint Louis: Mosby, 1984.

Tartaglia MG: Nursing diagnosis: Keystone of your care plan. *Nursing 85* 1985; 15: 3.

Yokom C: The differentiation of fear and anxiety. In Kim, McFarland, McLane (editors), *Classification of nursing diagnoses: Proceedings of the Fifth National Conference.* Saint Louis: Mosby, 1984.

Index

A

E

L

M

N

O

P

T

Addison-Wesley Health Sciences books are available at fine health sciences bookstores everywhere, but you may also order direct from us.

Please send _____ copies of the CARE PLANNING POCKET GUIDE #16305

_____ copies x $9.95 = (TOTAL AMOUNT) _____

☐ my check is enclosed

☐ bill my MasterCard   # _____ expiration date _____

☐ bill my Visa   # _____ expiration date _____

If your check accompanies your order, Addison-Wesley will ship your book/s free.

Billing address: _____
                    name
                    _____
                    address
                    _____
                    city/state/zip

Shipping address: _____
(if different)   name
                    _____
                    address
                    _____
                    city/state/zip

_____
authorized charge card signature

✳ ✳

Have you seen THE MANUAL OF NURSING THERAPEUTICS? It's the first portable guide to planning and evaluating adult care. It will help you to apply specific nursing diagnoses and interventions to more than 175 medical-surgical disorders. Written in a handy outline format, it includes the following for each disorder: brief review of pathophysiology; physical assessment data; diagnostic testing data; medical management and surgical interventions; nursing diagnoses and interventions specific to each disorder; outcome criteria and nursing interventions; patient-family teaching and discharge planning data. The handy spiral bound MANUAL was originated and developed by nurse and editor Pamela L. Swearingen, RN, with contributions from 23 expert clinicians. 590 pp., 1986

Please send me _____ copies of THE MANUAL OF NURSING THERA-PEUTICS #12940 at $19.95 and I'll pay as indicated above (_____ copies x $19.95 = _____)

Return this form to: Order Department, Addison-Wesley Publishing Company, One Jacob Way, Reading, MA 01867.

Prices indicated will be honored through June 1, 1987.